THE HAN┐ FO┐

HOSPITAL
CARE
ASSISTANTS
AND SUPPORT WORKERS

Edited by Lynne Swiatczak and Sue Benson

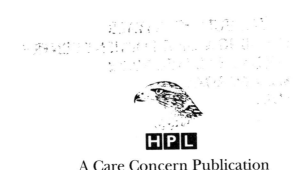

A Care Concern Publication

First published in 1993 by
Hawker Publications Ltd
13 Park House
140 Battersea Park Road
London SW11 4NB

British Library Cataloguing in Publication Data

A catalogue record for this book is available
from the British Library

ISBN 1 874790 10 8

Designed by
Richard Souper

Phototypeset by
Hawker Publications

Printed and bound in Great Britain by
Ipswich Book Co Ltd, Ipswich

Other titles in this series:
Handbook for Care Assistants – A Practical Guide to Caring for Elderly People
Third Edition (revised) 1993. ISBN 0 874790 06 X
The Care Assistant's Guide to Working With Elderly Mentally Infirm People
1991. ISBN 0 9514649 6 5
A Practical Guide to Working with People With Learning Disabilities
1992. ISBN 1 874790 00 0

Contents

Contributors

Rosemary Ashbee is manager of the Royal National Institute for the Blind's Westcliff House, Westgate-on-sea, Kent. She began her career as a care assistant with RNIB 13 years ago, and has trained in social work and communication with the deaf-blind.

Sue Benson BA RGN is editor of *Care Concern* books and educational materials, and editor of Dementia Care journal. She also works as a hospital "bank" nurse and lectures on the BTEC GNVQ course in Health and Social Care at Kingston College.

Karen Bryan PhD BSc MCSLT is a lecturer in acquired communication disorders at the National Hospitals College of Speech Sciences. She also works as a speech therapist with elderly people.

Stuart Darby BA RGN RMN RHV DPSN is Head of the Community Nursing Development Team within Camden and Islington Community Health Services NHS Trust. He is current chair of the Royal College of Nursing membership group FOCUS: On Older People, Nursing and Mental Health.

Anne Eaton RGN RM RCNT RNT Cert Ed is NVQ Coordinator at the Mid Trent College of Nursing and Midwifery. She teaches on NVQ courses at Levels 2 nd 3, and is an Internal Verifier and External Verifier for BTEC.

Peter Ferns is an Independent Training Consultant in the areas of learning disability, mental health and community care management issues. As a Black trainer he has been involved in many initiatives on race equality in care work.

Claire Hale BA PhD RGN RNT is a research associate at the Centre for Health Services Research at the University of Newcastle upon Tyne, and a senior nurse (research) at the Royal Victoria Hospital, Newcastle.

Wendy Hewitt-Sayer MN RGN RM Dip(N) is Director of Nursing and Quality Assurance, St Peter's Hospital NHS Trust, Chertsey, Surrey.

Ally Lallmahomed RMN RGN Dip(N) is Acting Nurse Manager of the Medical CMU, St. Peter's Hospital NHS Trust. He is currently undertaking an MSc in Research and Evaluation.

Sheila Mackie Bailey BA SRN RCNT DipNEd RNT is a freelance lecturer, consultant and author. Her interests include elderly people, nursing ethics and nursing research.

James Marr BA (Education) RGN RMN RCNT RNT is Consultant Nurse in the Nursing Development Unit for Older People, Tameside General Hospital, Lancashire. He is currently studying for an MA in gerontology.

Tim Martin RMN BSc (Nursing Studies) is Nursing Developments Officer for Salford Area Health Authority, Manchester.

Jane Maxim PhD MA DipCST MCSLT is a senior lecturer at the National Hospitals College of Speech Sciences. She is a speech therapist whose research area is language change in dementia, and she works with elderly stroke patients.

Esther Parker MN RGN RSCN NDN FEATC PGCEA RNT is Paediatric Nurse Tutor at the North West London College of Nursing and Midwifery.

Judith Roberts RGN RSCN Cert Health Ed, Cert Ed is Head of Unit, NVQs in Care, at Wirral Metropolitan College.

Lynn Sbaih BSc RGN RMN ENB199 (Accident and Emergency Nursing) is Senior Lecturer in Health Care Studies at Manchester Metropolitan University.

John Swiatczak RGN is a staff nurse on the Elderly Care Unit, Eaves Lane Hospital, Chorley, Lancashire.

Lynne Swiatczak RGN RNMH BSc is Directorate Manager, Services for Older People/Nursing Development Unit, Tameside General Hospital, Ashton-under-Lyne, Lancashire.

Kim Turner SRN RM ADM is Midwifery Manager, Community Services, St Peter's Hospital NHS Trust, Chertsey, and a Regional Representative for the Royal College of Midwives.

Michael Wafer BSc RGN, RNMH is Senior Nurse (Quality Assurance) at the Nursing Development Unit for Older People, Tameside Hospital, Lancashire.

Carol Welch RNMH RMN is a manager of nursing services with Fife Healthcare, responsible for nursing services to Lynebank Hospital and community teams for people with learning disabilities.

Helen White RGN RHV is continence adviser at the Dene Centre, Newcastle-upon-Tyne Council for the Disabled.

Margaret Whoriskey is a clinical psychologist with Fife Healthcare, working both in a hospital for people with learning disabilities and as a member of a multi-disciplinary community team.

Foreword

by Wilma MacPherson, Director of Quality and Nursing
Guy's and St Thomas' Hospital Trust, London

The end of the 1980s and the beginning of the 90s has seen an enormous change in the way in which nursing care is delivered in the health service.

This has resulted from the change in the role of student nurses. Traditionally a large part of direct patient care was delivered by nurses in training. With the advent of the Project 2000 scheme of training, much of the students' clinical experience is in a supervised supernumerary role. This of course has resulted in a vacuum in the care team, giving rise to the development of the care assistant/support worker role. As with any change, the nursing profession did not immediately see this as a potential opportunity in the delivery of patient care and was slow, I believe, to examine the full potential of the role that the care assistant could play in the team.

From hesitant beginnings, however, many examples of excellent practice are emerging in terms of the range and skills that such a person can add to the overall quality of patient care. At the same time as the need for this role was being identified vocational qualifications were beginning to be developed for the health care sector, enabling the emerging care assistant to attain National Vocational Qualifications commensurate with their role in care delivery.

This has brought its own set of challenges to the health service, since the competency-based approach to learning outcomes is not something that nurses have been accustomed to using in the preparation of student nurses. Coming to terms with this new way of carrying out assessment has brought its own set of headaches to many in an already overworked clinical team. Despite this, there have been many outstanding achievements by these men and women who have come into the health service by this route.

Recently we have been faced with the reduction in the hours that junior doctors work; an improvement which undoubtedly is long overdue. In analysing the activities that junior doctors were undertaking, we were able to identify an element of their work that could be carried out by appropriately trained care assistants in the future.

To this end, we began our first training programme of existing staff identified within the organisation from backgrounds as nursing auxiliaries, receptionists and ward clerks. The programme they embarked on equipped them to undertake elements of medical record keeping, phlebotomy, taking of ECGs as well as aspects of direct patient care in support of the nursing staff.

These workers have been trained to NVQ Level 3 mainly on a work based programme supported by day release and Open College material. Quite apart from the added value that their contribution is giving to the organisation, it has been noticeable from observing this group of staff that they have developed significantly as people, and are bringing valuable interest and excitement to the work they are doing.

The production of this book is most timely as the growing work of these new clinical team members is recognised and their role developed across a range of specialties. Appropriate literature to provide and support their new found learning is most welcome.

Acknowledgements

We would like to thank Anne Eaton, NVQ Coordinator at the Mid Trent College of Nursing and Midwifery, for compiling the lists of NVQ units covered in each chapter. Thanks also to the staff and patients of St Peter's Hospital, Chertsey, who appear in the photographs.

Introduction

As the role of the care assistant, support worker or nursing auxiliary on the hospital ward grows in importance and value to the caring team, so the need for training has increased. This book has been planned and written by experienced practising nurses who have responsibility for training care assistants in hospitals. Its chapters provide the framework for training in the practical care skills and underpinning knowledge required for National/Scottish Vocational Qualifications in Care, up to and beyond Level 2 in Direct Care. It also covers useful material for other endorsements and in many cases goes beyond the requirements of Level 2, well on the way towards Level 3.

Practical instruction and work experience remain the cornerstones of training. This book's function is to add an extra dimension of knowledge, and the resources to question and challenge some of the practices, assumptions and attitudes care assistants are bound to meet.

Units of care related to NVQ/SVQs are very difficult to separate. No units can be fully covered in a book because the qualification must be practice-based and the units applied to individual care environments. It is vital, therefore, that care assistants liaise and discuss their progress, assessment and underpinning knowledge thoroughly and repeatedly with their work-based assessors, so that specific targets for acquiring and developing skills and knowledge can be identified and achieved. The main NVQ/SVQ units covered in each chapter are listed at the chapter's end.

We have decided, for simplicity, to use the term *care assistant* throughout the book, to include health support workers, nursing auxiliaries and any other title that describes the same role. We have also largely used the term *patients* to describe people in hospital care, except in the areas of mental health and learning disability, where the term *clients* is more commonly used.

To be of practical use as a handbook, we have felt it important that the book didn't grow too large and unwieldy. So we have decided, for example, not to attempt to cover the practicalities of First Aid and resuscitation, which depend not only on training but supervised practice, and in which all hospitals provide induction training and frequent updates for all staff. Other areas of care, notably lifting and handling patients, also depend on practical sessions, but are so much part of the care assistant's daily work that we felt it essential to include guidelines as a reminder and reinforcement of practical training.

Lynne Swiatczak and Sue Benson

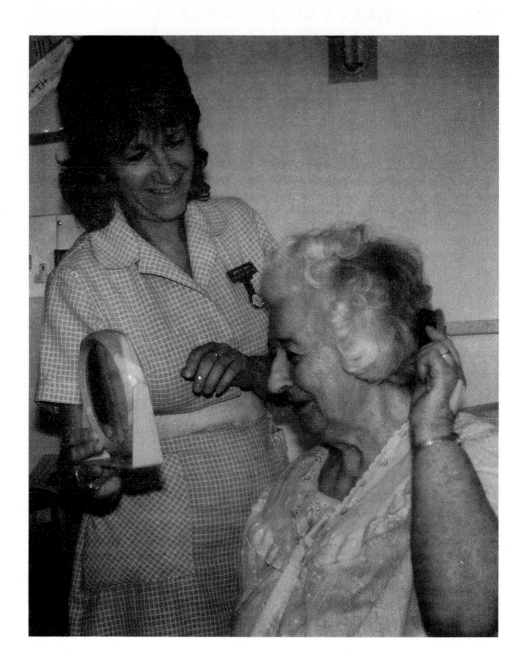

CHAPTER 1

The role of the care assistant

Lynne Swiatczak

*• Where care assistants work and what they do • Induction training
• Your place in the multidisciplinary team • How care is organised • Care plans
and your role in the delivery of care*

Care assistants in hospitals may work in any one of several different areas, in each of which their role will be different. But underlying the differences is the same basic role, examined in this chapter. I will also look at the various ways care is organised.

Hospitals can be awesome places, with numerous people in different uniforms wandering about, all looking as though they know what they are doing! As a new care assistant you may feel that you are the only one who is nervous. Understanding your role may help and this chapter will give information which may be helpful now and in the future.

Each ward, even within the same area, will have its own method of organisation and its own expectations of the care assistant. Although job/role descriptions are issued before employment, these are only outlines of the role and there may be many other aspects which you don't understand when you start work.

Induction courses

All hospitals should provide an induction course for new employees; this usually covers the following basic subjects together with specific information about the hospital:

• Fire safety and evacuation procedures
• Lifting and handling instruction
• Resuscitation and basic first aid
• Customer care training
• Health and safety in the workplace
• Occupational health information
• Sickness and absence reporting
• Payment information

In addition to the above, many units and wards provide their own induction courses which cover aspects specific to their needs.

On the ward

The ward sister or charge nurse will usually allocate a new care assistant to an experienced member of staff for the first few weeks or months of their employment in order for them to learn the "routine" of the ward.

To begin with, you will need to find out where the fire points are, what telephone number to dial for cardiac arrest, fire or emergency, what security arrangements are in force, how to report sick, arrangements for meals and payment details.

The ward sister or charge nurse will explain **policies and procedures** to the care assistant. An example would be the lifting policy and procedure, which documents the correct way to assess, plan and undertake a lift or transfer. Copies of these are usually kept in a prominent place on the ward and all members of staff must familiarise themselves with them.

The ward may also have its own set of **standards** which must be maintained and these will also be kept in a prominent place on the ward. Standards are documents which state the quality of care which will be given in that particular area. They usually cover areas such as record keeping and general ward facilities, and can cover specific areas such as communication and direct care giving (see example on page 135). Standards will reflect the philosophy of the ward and will be reviewed regularly.

The ward **philosophy** is also spelled out in a document which states the beliefs and values of the ward and its team. It should be readily available for staff and patients to see at any time.

The nursing team

The ward nursing team usually consists of the following staff:
• Senior sister or charge nurse
• Junior sister or charge nurse (in some wards this post may not be used)
• Staff nurses (these are nurses registered in either general nursing, mental illness, mental handicap or midwifery)
• Enrolled nurses (these nurses are second level registered nurses in the above areas)
• Learner nurses (studying the above areas; they are not on every ward)

• Care assistants (also called health care support workers or nursing auxiliaries).

This team will work together to provide the nursing care which each patient requires during his or her stay in hospital.

Ways of delivering care

Each ward will follow its own method of nursing and of organising the delivery of care to the patients. Within most hospitals in Great Britain there are four main methods used; these are changed according to the needs of particular areas of care or patient groups.

Task allocation

One of the oldest methods of delivering care is now little used as it does not provide the "holistic" or "whole person" approach to care which is encouraged today. However, "task allocation" is still used in some areas.

This system breaks down total patient care into a series of tasks which are then delegated by the person in charge to the rest of the ward team. This may mean that one nurse bathes a patient, another serves his meal, another carries out his wound care, another dispenses his medication etc. While this system effectively deals with the "work", it provides little opportunity for the patient to form any relationship with the people caring for them and also makes it difficult to provide a consistent approach to care.

Team nursing

The second method, commonly used, is "team nursing". In this method the ward staff are formed into teams, and each team cares for a group of patients while they are on duty. There is a team leader, usually a staff nurse or sister/charge nurse, who allocates work

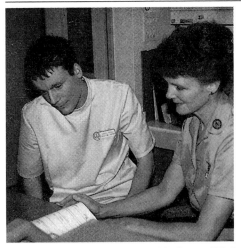

Working as part of the team with the qualified nurse – care plans must be followed exactly.

to the rest of the team for that shift or span of duty. This system means that the patients are nursed by the same small team of nurses and they are able to establish a relationship with them. It also means that their care can be communicated to the rest of the team easily, enabling all staff to be consistent. This system works best when the teams keep the same group of patients on each shift.

Patient allocation

The third method used is similar to team nursing and is called "patient allocation". In this system a number of patients are allocated to each nurse, who plans their care and together with other staff delivers the care to the patients. The nurse may keep the same patients for a long period of time or only for a span of duty. This system provides some continuity and allows relationships to be established. It also enables the patient to have a "named nurse" who is responsible for them.

Primary nursing

The fourth method, increasingly being used, is "primary nursing". This system involves each patient being allocated to a nurse for the whole of their stay on the ward, that is from admission to discharge.

The primary nurse is a registered nurse who works with an associate nurse and care assistant to provide all the care needed for the small group of patients allocated to them. The primary nurse is the "named nurse", who plans, gives and evaluates the care for each patient in the group. He or she is also responsible for communicating that care to the rest of the staff in order that care can be consistent. This system also encourages closer working with the patient and their family.

The care assistant has a role in each of these systems. The ward sister or charge nurse will explain which is used and what your specific role will be.

Care planning

Care planning is normally the role of the nurse responsible for the patient's care. A care plan is a document produced by the nurse together with the patient, which states how the patient is to be cared for. It will cover all areas of care – such as hygiene, continence, dressing, pain relief – and enables all who care for the patient to provide consistent, individual care.

Care plans should be read by all staff who are to provide care for the patient, and must be followed exactly. Care assistants do not plan care but can write in the care plan any care which they have provided.

The multidisciplinary team

The ward team will also include other people, who are known as members of the "multidisciplinary team". This means that all those who provide care or a specific service to the patient may be included under one heading. The most common members of the multi-disciplinary team are as follows:

Consultant: the physician or surgeon who is in charge of the patient's medical care.

Junior doctors: known by various titles and varying in seniority – there may be Registrars, Senior House Officers, House Officers, etc.

Physiotherapists provide a range of active and passive exercise programmes and treatments for individual patients.

Occupational therapists provide therapy based around activities of daily living, such as dressing, and assess how people will manage at home.

Dietitians provide dietary advice together with nutritional assessments and feeding advice, and formulate dietary supplements.

Speech therapists provide advice and treatment for speech problems and are also involved in helping patients with swallowing difficulties.

Pharmacists dispense the appropriate medication for patients and also give advice about medication to both patients and staff.

Chiropodists give advice and treatment for all patients with foot problems.

Social workers, discharge co-ordinators and others provide assessment and advice on numerous problems relating to discharge, home circumstances and benefits.

There are many other members of the multidisciplinary team, and care assistants will come into contact with most of them during their employment.

Specialist departments such x-ray, scanning or the dental department, all have their own specialist workers. The care assistant will come into contact with most of these at some time.

Other members of staff with whom the care assistant will have regular contact include domestic assistants, porters, laundry services and catering staff.

Caring for individuals

The main contact for all care assistants will, of course, be the patients. Each patient must be treated as an individual and each will have different needs. The type of condition which has brought the patient to hospital will decide which ward they are admitted to. Care assistants in almost all areas will give direct care to patients under the supervision of qualified nurses.

This care will range from greeting a patient on admission to carrying out last offices on patients who have died. It will also include washing and dressing patients, assisting with eating and drinking, mobility and lifting, and various other duties, some of which may be of an intimate nature. The care assistant must remember to provide privacy and protect the patient's dignity at all times, and must remain courteous throughout any care-giving activity.

There will also be other more general duties, which may include sorting and stacking linen and patients' clothing, making tea and coffee, serving meals, making beds and general ward tidying.

The care assistant may also be involved in other duties for which there will be specific training, for example taking routine observations of temperature, pulse, respiration and blood pressure, testing patients' urine samples or writing in patients' notes.

It is important that all staff carry out

only those duties for which they have received training and in which they feel competent. Some duties are restricted to qualified nurses and medical staff, and care assistants must ensure that they always act within their role description. This is necessary not only for the safety of patients but also for your benefit. Never be afraid to say you don't know and never be afraid to ask!

Escort duties

Care assistants are sometimes involved in escorting patients to different departments within the hospital and, on occasion, to other hospitals for specific tests or referrals.

The patient's condition must be stable and the care assistant should know the patient and feel confident to escort him or her. The relevant notes and/or documentation must be taken and the care assistant must know the department to be attended and the arrangements for transportation there and back. You must also have had training in basic first aid and know how to summon help in an emergency.

In many cases the patient's anxiety and stress can be reduced if they are accompanied by a care assistant they know.

Lifting and transferring

One of the main areas of care in adult areas is assisting patients with transfer and change of position. This may include a range of activities, from positioning a walking frame near to the patient to physically lifting them from bed to chair.

All staff must have appropriate training in manual handling regulations and techniques before they attempt to move any patient. This is for the benefit of the staff as well as patients, as back injuries can mean an end to your career. Moving and lifting, a very important aspect of the care assistant's role, is covered in Chapter 7 of this book.

A varied role

You can see from this chapter that the role of the care assistant is varied. It is also very important in the provision of good quality care to patients. Care assistants must always work within the bounds of their role description and capabilities. I hope you will find your chosen work rewarding and satisfying.

Points to remember

1. If you are unsure, always ask!
2. Always follow the policies and procedures of the ward and/or hospital.
3. Always read the patient's care plan before giving any care, and follow it exactly.

NVQ Levels 2 & 3 Value Base Units
Oc Promote and support individual rights and choice within service delivery.
Oe Support individuals through effective communication.

Levels 2 & 3 Core Units
U4 Contribute to the health, safety and security of individuals and their environment.
U5 Obtain, transmit and store information relating to the delivery of a care service.
W3 Support clients in transition due to their care requirements.

Level 2 Direct Care Endorsement
Z7 Contribute to the movement and treatment of clients to maximise their physical comfort.

CHAPTER 2

Your responsibilities

Lynne Swiatczak

• Your responsibility as a member of the caring team • Confidentiality Health and safety • Resuscitation • Dispensing medication, and wound care • Written records • Complaints • Taking telephone messages • Customer relations • Reporting bad practice

As a care assistant you have a number of responsibilities to your patients and to your employers. There are several areas of responsibility which have a direct effect on the care of individual patients, including confidentiality, health and safety, resuscitation and dispensing medication. Others have an indirect effect: these include documentation (written records), complaints, telephone messages, customer relations and reporting bad practice.

Each of these areas will be covered in this chapter, but remember that each hospital will have its own policies and procedures – these are not standard throughout hospitals. All staff, whether qualified or unqualified, must become familiar with these policies and procedures as soon as possible and, if in doubt, must ask advice before giving information or taking part in any practice they are uncertain about.

Confidentiality

This area is of the utmost priority. All patients have the right to have information about themselves and their condition kept confidential. Only those people to whom the patient gives permission have the right of access to that information.

Within hospitals it is accepted that nurses, doctors and other members of the multi-disciplinary team have access to information about patients, and they will write in the patient's medical and nursing notes. This only relates to the patients within their care, however.

The patient must also be informed of any local policies which affect confidentiality, for example access to nursing notes. Some hospitals give patients open access to their nursing notes and keep them in different places on the ward, usually at the bedside. This can affect confidentiality as the notes cannot be kept under watch at all times and relatives/carers and other staff on the ward may be able to read them. If a system like this is in place, the consequences must be fully discussed with the patient before notes are left with them.

Every qualified nurse is bound by a Code of Conduct which has specific guidance on confidentiality. Care assistants as a group are not bound by such a code, but some hospitals have their own policy regarding confidentiality and unqualified staff. An example of a policy for confidentiality is as follows; it gives a brief outline of responsibility in this area:

• The care assistant must not divulge any confidential information to police, media, relatives, carers or other disciplines unless otherwise informed by the qualified nurse responsible for the patient's care.

• Information given to the care assistant must be passed on to the qualified nurse if this information relates to the patient's treatment. If in doubt the information must be passed to the qualified nurse, who will decide how to deal with the information.

• As far as possible the permission of the patient should be gained before giving confidential information to anyone else.

• The care assistant must not disclose any information about patients to any person outside the hospital. This also includes discussing patients with other staff where conversation may be overheard.

This last point may seem obvious, but it is one of the most important. All staff working with patients must remember that it is not appropriate to discuss patients at all when they are not on the ward. This includes other wards in the hospital, the dining room etc, where conversation can be overheard.

Health and safety

The Health and Safety at Work Act 1974 affects every employee including those in hospitals. The Act makes it everyone's responsibility to report any hazard in the work area and to ensure they are aware of all safety regulations which may apply.

Health and safety at work is normally covered during the induction course when a new employee starts work. Most hospitals also provide annual updates for all staff. Safety representatives are appointed by Trade Unions; all staff should find out who their representative is and how they can be contacted.

Each piece of equipment on wards must be checked regularly and should also have its operating instructions attached to it. Never use a piece of equipment if you have not been instructed in its use. This can be dangerous not only for the patient but also for yourself.

Health and safety also relates to areas such as food hygiene and storage, cleanliness of ward areas, first aid training and fire instruction. All employees should follow policies and procedures correctly.

The occupational health department of each hospital will provide health education and advice and is also available to provide treatment should staff require this while at work. This department is also involved in accident prevention, particularly needlestick injuries and back problems.

Resuscitation

Each hospital will have its own policy regarding the role of the care assistant in resuscitation of patients. This can range from summoning help to actively taking part in the resuscitation procedure.

The least which will be expected of the care assistant will be to know how to summon help, where the emergency equipment is kept and how to deal with relatives/carers who may be present. This is an extremely important role, particularly in areas where there are few qualified nurses, as the care assistant will be relied on to carry out these duties, leaving the qualified nurse free to actively resuscitate the patient.

If the care assistant is needed to participate more fully, they will require further training and assessment. The resuscitation procedure consists of artificially ventilating the patient (getting air into the lungs) and carrying out cardiac massage (assisting the heart to pump blood around the body). Both of these are areas where the care assistant may be involved.

A cardiac arrest is a stressful event for all staff, and it is important that everyone is fully equipped to carry out their part in the procedure. If in doubt ask; do not attempt to assist if you are unsure as this can cause more problems.

First Aid

First Aid will be covered in your induction course and most hospitals provide annual update sessions for all staff. First Aid courses usually cover nosebleeds, wounds, broken bones, burns and scalds, and shock.

Dispensing medication

In most hospitals, qualified nurses dispense medication to patients on their own. This is accepted by the UKCC (the governing body of registered nurses). There are still some areas however, which use two nurses. These are usually one qualified and one learner, but may be one qualified and one care assistant. There will be specific local policies regarding the dispensing of medication to patients, and these must be strictly followed.

The usual role for the care assistant will be to give the medicines to the patient when they have been dispensed by the nurse, and the patient's identity has been checked to ensure that the

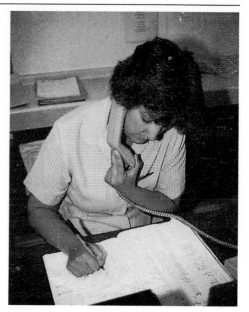

When you answer the telephone be ready to speak – don't keep the caller waiting.

right patient receives the right drug. The nurse checks the patient's identity by either asking the patient their name and/or checking the patient's identity band which carries their name and hospital number.

The patient must be seen to take their medication; if they refuse, the medication must be removed and the omission noted. Patients must not be left with medication and it should never be left on lockers and bed tables where it could be taken by other patients.

Care assistants do not normally give injections; this procedure should be carried out by a qualified nurse although help may be required to position the patient.

Wound care

In some areas care assistants are involved in dressing patients' wounds. If this is required then training and assessment will be given, and procedures which are

18

documented on the ward must be followed. It is important that the patient has the correct dressing and that aseptic principles are followed in order to prevent infection occurring. (Aseptic principles ensure that as far as possible the dressing is done under sterile or scrupulously clean conditions.)

Documentation

In some hospitals the care assistant is expected to document – record in writing – the care they have given, in the patient's nursing notes. The information documented is usually restricted to recording what has been carried out, as the planning of care is the province of the qualified nurse.

Each hospital which uses this system will have guidelines which should be followed at all times. The signature of the care assistant will normally be countersigned by the qualified nurse in charge of the patient's care.

Documentation is also required if care assistants are involved in carrying out observations such as temperature and blood pressure. These must be recorded on the appropriate chart and must be reported to the nurse in charge of the patient's care if they are outside the normal limits for the patient.

Complaints

Complaints can come from a variety of sources. A patient may complain; it may be their relative/carer, another nurse, doctor or members of staff from another department. All complaints must be dealt with according to the hospital's complaints procedure, and staff should make sure they are aware of the relevant policies to be followed.

There are several points usually found in complaints procedures, as follows:

• Always treat every complaint seriously.

• Always pass a complaint (whether written or verbal) to the person in charge of the ward or department.

• Always listen to the person making a complaint. Do not interrupt.

• Never assume that the person is getting at you personally.

• Never assume that the person has got the facts wrong.

• Always stay cool and calm and try to get all the facts.

• Never argue with the person making the complaint.

Usually the complaint will be dealt with by the person in charge of the ward or department. You may, however, be required to make a statement regarding the complaint. You can ask for advice on how to do this from your Trade Union representative, or help can be made available from the hospital legal department.

If **you** wish to complain, similar principles apply. You should complain through the nurse in charge of the ward or department:

• Be specific and give the time and date that the incident happened.

• Be courteous and polite but firm and confident.

• Complain verbally first. If nothing happens, put your complaint in writing and keep a copy of the letter.

Telephone messages

There are several points to note when taking telephone messages. Each hospital will have its own specific guidelines, but some points are standard:

• When you answer the telephone always be ready to speak immediately, do not keep the caller waiting.

• Always give a greeting, the ward or department name, your name and full title and ask the caller if you can help them.

• If you cannot help then be sure to put the caller in touch with someone who can.

• You must be able to use your hospital telephone system and know how to transfer calls.

• The most important point to remember is always to pass on messages to patients, relatives or members of staff.

Customer relations

The patients are your customers. There are also staff from other departments who may be your customers. There are several points to remember when dealing with anyone in your working day:

• Treat others as you would like to be treated yourself.

• Listen to your customer and do not allow your attention to wander.

• Try to see things from the customer's point of view.

• Make sure you are polite, courteous and helpful.

• Look as well as listen; pick up non-verbal cues such as gestures and facial expressions.

It is important that you always make the patient feel as though you have time for them, even if you are busy. Patients' needs are important and you must find time for them.

Reporting bad practice

This is a very important responsibility, not only for the care assistant but for all staff. The patients must at all times receive care of the highest standard; they should never be mistreated either deliberately or by negligence on the part of staff.

In most areas the care given will be of the highest standards and the patients will suffer no harm. It is important, however, that staff are aware of how to report bad practice or abuse and that this is done immediately in order to protect the patient.

In many areas staff will have to deal with difficult situations where patients are potentially violent. Aggression should never be met with aggression; most situations can be defused if staff remain calm and soothing. Try to keep the patient calm; do not raise your voice or argue. Patients who are physically aggressive should never be hit by any member of staff; self defence is not an excuse.

If the situation is dangerous then alternative action should be taken. Leaving the situation is better for both staff and patient, and often it is wiser for the care assistant to summon assistance if a situation is difficult, than to deal with it themselves.

If a member of staff is seen physically or verbally abusing a patient this must be reported to the person in charge of the ward/department immediately. Never try to deal with the situation yourself, it is inappropriate and could result in disciplinary action for yourself if you do not report the occurrence.

There are other examples of bad practice which are equally important: patients who need positional changes but are left in one position for long periods of time; patients who are left in wet clothing and bedclothes; patients who are ignored when they ask for help – all these are examples of bad practice and each member of staff has a responsibility to ensure that none of these happens to their patients.

Each hospital will also have policies on

restraint and these should be fully understood by all staff. Patients should not be restrained as a general rule, and it is not acceptable to place patients in situations from which they have no escape.

Remember that if you see it and allow it to happen you are as guilty. Many Trade Unions have methods by which people can report things anonymously and if this is the only option then it should be taken; someone must be told.

Varied responsibilities

As can be seen from the information in this chapter, the responsibilities of the care assistant are many and varied. The qualified nurse in charge of the ward or department accepts responsibility on behalf of the staff although staff are still accountable for their own actions. It is very important that care assistants follow hospital policies and procedures fully and that they are trained to carry out these procedures.

Legally the hospital as your employer will normally accept "vicarious liability" on your behalf. This means that if you were sued for an incident which occurred whilst you were working they would accept responsibility on your behalf and would provide a defence for you.

This only applies, however, if you were following the policies laid down by the hospital at that time. Ignorance of these policies is no defence and it is your responsibility to make sure you are familiar with them as soon as possible after you start employment.

Throughout your work your main responsibility is to give the best possible care to your patients at all times. If you are unable to do this through problems such as lack of staff or facilities then you should bring this to the attention of the person in charge of the ward or department immediately, so that they can deal with the problem.

Points to remember

1. Always treat your patients the way you would wish to be treated yourself.
2. Always follow policies and procedures correctly.
3. Always maintain the patient's confidentiality.
4. Always use equipment correctly.
5. Always pass on messages promptly and accurately.
6. Never accept bad practice.

NVQ Levels 2 & 3 Value Base Units
Oa Promote anti-discriminatory practice.
Ob Maintain confidentiality of information.
Oc Promote and support individual rights and choice within service delivery.
Od Acknowledge individuals' personal beliefs and identity.
Oe Support individuals through effective communication.

Levels 2 & 3 Core Units
U5 Obtain, transmit and store information relating to the delivery of a care service.
U4 Contribute to the health, safety and security of individuals and their care environment.

CHAPTER 3

Talking and listening

Jane Maxim and Karen Bryan

*• How to convey information clearly and be a good listener
• Using your eyes as well as your ears • Different ways of speaking • Language
barriers • How being ill in hospital affects communication • Problems following
surgery • Stroke and language disorders • Elderly people • Dementia
• Mental illness • Learning disability • Talking to children
• How to help people with hearing problems*

What is communication? What can make communication difficult for somebody who is in hospital? What can be done to make communication easier?

These questions all use the term communication. It is often said that someone is a good communicator when they can talk well and interest their listener. But there are two sides to good communication: being able to make the meaning clear **and** being able to listen and understand what is being said.

For most people, good communication is an important part of their daily life. For people who are ill in hospital away from their families, perhaps restricted to bed and very anxious about their illness, their operation or the progress of their recovery, communication is particularly important.

As well as conveying their needs and asking questions, many people in hospital will welcome the opportunity to talk about their worries. They will also want to hear and to talk about what is happening outside the restricted environment of the hospital ward.

Look and listen

Communication is the process of conveying information between two or more people. Communication involves talking, listening, writing and reading, facial expression, gesture and body language. Thoughts are put into words and sentences to convey meaning. Speech is produced by co-ordinated muscle movements of the larynx, tongue and face. But part of the message is conveyed by other means:

• hand and body movements to produce gestures such as shrugging the shoulders
• changes in voice and pitch, for example we describe someone as "sounding" angry
• the use of facial expression such as a smile or frown.

The listener needs to listen to the actual words spoken **and** attend to the other information that the speaker is conveying, in order to fully appreciate the meaning. So listening involves using your eyes as well as your ears.

Different ways of speaking
People vary tremendously in the way they

speak. Men sound different from women and people have a wide range of different accents (the way we speak) and dialects (what words we use and the way we use them). In addition, we all vary the way we speak depending on who we are speaking to and the circumstances of the conversation. Most of the time we do this without even being aware of it.

To take an example, the way in which we speak to a colleague at work is very different to the way in which we speak to a baby or young child. With a colleague we have a shared knowledge of the job to be done and use the appropriate vocabulary for that situation. We are speaking to someone whom we assume will understand what we are saying without any need for us to change the way we speak. However, if we were explaining part of the job to somebody who was not familiar with it, then the type and amount of information we give would vary.

It is important that when you talk to patients in hospital, you give them the right amount of information: too little and they will not understand you, too much and they will feel that you are treating them as if they are stupid.

It is also important not to assume that people who are ill or in some way disabled are automatically incapable of normal understanding and speaking. The people you will encounter in hospital may have differing styles of speech. Some people have very quiet

- **Be sensitive to the different ways in people speak.**

- **Be aware of how you are speaking yourself.**

- **Don't jump to hasty assumptions about people just because of the way they sound.**

voices, others very loud ones, someone may be used to speaking in short, abrupt phrases while other people may talk at great length with lots of detail.

Language barriers

Most people have experienced difficulty in communicating while on holiday in another country. A simple task such as buying a railway ticket can become almost impossible when two people do not speak, understand, read or write the same language.

There are many people in Britain who live within communities where little or in some cases no English is spoken. When someone who speaks little or no English comes into hospital, they have all the factors associated with their illness to cope with, as well as difficulty in communicating.

In order to make communication easier:

- watch the person's facial expression and gestures as these may convey some of the meaning

- try to anticipate their needs, for example by looking around their bed and on their locker to see if anything is wrong

- speak to the person in a normal voice at a normal speed, but use short sentences and attempt to convey only the important points

- use gestures as you speak, for example "Do you want a drink?" can be accompanied by a mime of drinking

- try to find out about the person from their family or friends, who may be able to help by writing down some key words for you with a translation, and can tell you a little about the person, the way they are feeling and any particular dislikes they may have

- if the person has no visitors, try to find a

• **Communication difficulty leads to immense frustration.**

• **It often gains the person the label of being "difficult"**

• **Communication difficulty can also affect relationships with other people, including family and friends, and can lead to social isolation.**

member of staff or even another patient in the hospital who can speak the same language. Most hospitals have a list of staff who speak other languages.

How illness affects us

Imagine how you might feel in hospital: lonely, very unsure about what is happening, worrying about what will happen next, feeling ill, uncomfortable, or in pain. All these factors are bound to affect the way a person communicates with others.

Some people may react by being over-cheerful and trying to convince everyone else that they are not at all worried; others may become very quiet and withdrawn; others may be abstracted and so appearing to not really know what is happening; others may be very forceful and angry, perhaps about trivial things. Therefore it is important to think about why a person may speak to you in a way that you don't expect.

Added to the effect of being in hospital is the variation in communication discussed in the section above. All this means that you must try to:

• approach patients carefully in a sensitive manner

• react calmly to the patient

• be sympathetic to their situation

• have some understanding of why the patient may react oddly.

As well as all of the factors mentioned above, many patients in hospital may have specific difficulties in communicating. All the problems described in the following sections of this chapter will affect the ability of people in hospital to communicate normally. It is important to consider the impact on a person of not being able to communicate normally. It will lead to:

• difficulty in expressing immediate wants, for example to go to the toilet

• difficulty in expressing feelings such as sadness, anger

• difficulty in expressing needs, for example to see a particular member of their family.

After surgery

A person who has just returned to a hospital ward may be affected by some or all of the following factors:

• The effects of the anaesthetic may still be evident making them very sleepy, not very responsive. Their voice may be very quiet or even hoarse and their speech rather indistinct or slurred.

• Drugs such as pain killers or sedatives may have similar effects. Occasionally drugs can make a person feel irritable or even aggressive.

• The person may be feeling pain, discomfort or nausea.

Confusion

Due to a combination of these factors, the person may be partly or completely confused. "Confusion" refers to a change in a person's mental state which shows itself in:

• reduced recognition, understanding of and response to the environment

• difficulty with recent and distant memory

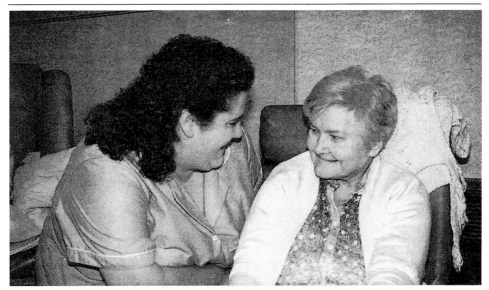

When talking to someone suffering from dementia, keep it direct with no unnecessary details.

• inability to think clearly

• disorientation to time, place and person, where the person is unsure of where they are, how long they have been there and who they are with.

What the person says may therefore not make complete sense as it reflects these difficulties. As the effects of drugs and anaesthesia wear off, the confusion will gradually decrease. The person may need to be helped out of confusion by talking about what has happened and where they are. The person will need lots of reassurance and encouragement to help them to start communicating appropriately again.

Other patients who are not so severely affected may still be slightly mixed up about very recent events, such as what happened just before or just after their operation. They may also be emotionally very sensitive. They may cry very easily or get cross or even angry about something that would not usually cause such a strong reaction – for example being asked if they would like to sit up.

Anxiety and embarrassment

Anxiety or worry can obviously cause a person to react in an unexpected way. Embarrassment can also lead to this. A previously independent person may be very embarrassed by needing help with, for example, toileting. Privacy is often very limited on a hospital ward, which can contribute to embarrassment.

It is important that although *you* have become used to the hospital routines, you do not forget that these can be strange or even seem degrading to some patients. It is therefore important to explain what is being done and why, and to understand the reasons why a patient might be unco-operative or even get angry with you.

Anger and abuse

A patient who is angry may even show this by shouting at you, possibly by verbal abuse such as swearing and especially if he or she has difficulty in talking, by trying to push you away or even throwing something towards you.

Remember to remain calm and try to

> **Coping with anger:**
> • **accept that the person is expressing strong feelings and do not try to contradict or belittle these feelings**
> • **give the person a chance to discuss how they are feeling and what is really upsetting them so that you can try to understand the situation**
> • **speak calmly and gently and offer reassurance once the outburst is over**

understand what is happening. Often the person has been gradually becoming more frustrated, perhaps by their restricted mobility, or maybe they are really upset because their family have not yet visited. Or perhaps they have just been told bad news about their medical condition.

Stroke

Patients may come into hospital because they have had a stroke, but there are also a large number of people who have survived a stroke and who subsequently enter hospital for another reason. These people may still have residual problems from the original stroke, such as difficulty in communicating.

Dysphasia
Stroke can damage certain areas of the brain which cause an adult to have an acquired language disorder, called dysphasia. In dysphasia the ability to understand and express meaning through words is disrupted. This may affect speech, reading and writing.

The exact effect of a stroke on speech and language will vary from one individual to another depending upon their injury, their previous education, work and experiences, their personality and their present communication needs relating to their environment.

Dysphasic adults may have non-fluent speech: they have difficulty producing sentences or even words in severe cases. For example, they might say "doctor" where "I would like to see the doctor" might be expected, or "wu" for water.

Sometimes errors are made. These may involve changing sounds – "ted" for "bed" – or use of an incorrect word – "boy" for "girl". Other dysphasic people may have fluent speech but difficulty in finding the right words. For example:

"That's a, oh a, you know, tea, tea, drink it, no *cup*".

In other cases, although speech is fluent, it is not correctly structured so that little meaning is expressed.

A person's understanding of language can also be disrupted by dysphasia but not necessarily in the same way as their expressive speech. Reading and writing are usually affected in the same way as speech, but occasionally someone is able to write down what they cannot say.

Where possible a speech and language therapist can be asked to give details of a dysphasic person's speech and language abilities and to give specific advice on the most effective ways of achieving communication. Staff and carers can also observe a dysphasic person, noting the difficulties that they are having with communication and what helps them with this.

The following general guidelines are helpful to remember when speaking to a dysphasic person:

• Slow down.

• Remove distractions (eg TV).

• Break any speech into stages. For example :

"It's getting cold, isn't it?"
"Are you cold?"
"Do you want a blanket?"

• Try to understand the person. Asking questions which only need a yes/no answer may help to give you clues. For example "Is it sore?"

• Maintain contact with the person while they struggle to speak: look towards them, look interested and wait patiently.

• Give them time to speak.

• Commiserate with them if they become upset or frustrated.

• The person is not stupid; speaking loudly and slowly does not help. Use normal voice and expression.

• Ask the person's opinion.

• Use gesture – "Would you like a cup of coffee?" – point to the coffee pot while asking.

• Try to remember that speaking and understanding may be a great effort, so try to break up taking a case history etc. Do not expect a dysphasic person to talk for too long, and be alert to signs of fatigue.

> **Dysphasia is a language disorder which may affect understanding, speaking, reading and writing.**
>
> **Dysarthria is a speech disorder caused by poor muscle movement or poor muscle coordination.**

Dysarthria

Problems with physically producing the sounds of speech can also occur after stroke and some other diseases such as Parkinson's disease, multiple sclerosis, and motor neurone disease.

This is called dysarthria and refers to a difficulty in speech production with no problems in understanding, reading or writing (unless another physical problem, such as arthritic fingers, affects these).

The main forms of dysarthria are:

Flaccid dysarthria: Here the muscles are weak and floppy. The person may have a very quiet voice making them sound difficult to hear, and their speech may sound unclear.

Spastic dysarthria: Here the muscles are very stiff, making movement difficult. Speech is therefore jerky with sudden changes in loudness.

Parkinsonian dysarthria: Here the muscles are stiff and unco-ordinated. This causes the person's speech to speed up, and the speech is often difficult to hear at the end of a sentence.

A person with dysarthria can understand language fully and has no problem in thinking what to say or in formulating a response in his head, but has a physical difficulty in speaking the words because the speech muscles are not working normally.

In some cases very little speech can be achieved, or the speech is unintelligible. However, it is often the case that people in everyday contact with a dysarthric speaker can "tune in" to their speech and understand them well. Some dysarthric people are able to use writing or a communication aid such as a pointing chart or an electronic device, to add to or replace their speech.

Elderly people

Elderly people essentially speak and understand in the same way as younger people. They may suffer from sensory losses such as reduced vision and hearing which can be corrected provided that glasses and hearing aids are worn. Teeth are also important for speech, so if dentures are used they should always be worn and should be regularly checked to ensure that they fit correctly.

However, research shows that elderly people hesitate and pause more when

> **Is the elderly person**
> • **wearing cleaned glasses?**
> • **wearing a hearing aid in good working order?**
> • **wearing dentures that fit well?**

they speak. Older people say themselves that they sometimes find it difficult to remember a particular word, often a name. But everyone has this difficulty from time to time. Elderly people may also be *slower* at understanding what is said to them, although their actual ability to understand is not diminished. It is important therefore that hospital staff speak to older people as they would to younger adults. There is a tendency to speak to older people as if they are small children, which should be avoided.

Elderly people may of course suffer from specific diseases that can affect their ability to talk and understand in the same way as younger people.

Dementia

Unfortunately, a minority of elderly people suffer from **dementia**, a gradual loss of brain cells resulting in progressive loss of memory, slowing of activity and difficulty with the tasks of everyday life. Communication is also affected in dementia.

As the disease progresses, communication is affected by memory loss, and the ability to name people and objects is gradually reduced. The fluency of speech increases so that speech becomes rambling and fragmented. Here is an example from an eighty-two year old lady with a two-year history of dementia, describing a picture of a busy high street. She has been widowed for twenty years:

"Two ladies, baker, somebody leading a little baby. I had a little baby. I don't see much of my husband now. She turned around and looked at me. Supermarket".

Understanding becomes gradually more difficult and there may be problems with reading and writing.

In the later stages of dementia, speech reduces until the person only speaks occasional words. Some people also produce echo-speech, repeating what has been said to them. By this stage the person has severe problems with understanding and is probably only able to understand a few conversational points. Reading and writing become impossible.

It is obviously difficult to communicate with a person suffering from advanced dementia. However, the early and middle stages can last for many years, and during this time effective communication can be achieved.

There are five basic points to consider in order to assist communication with someone who is suffering from dementia:

1. Do not assume that any aspects of meaning which are not specified will be understood. For example, you may talk about the next meal and be very well aware that this must be breakfast because it is 7am and the elderly person is just getting up. But you must make this clear, by using the word "breakfast".

2. Be very direct – cut out any unnecessary details.

3. Keep the content direct. For example, the remark "I imagine it's rather like flying" would be very difficult for a dementia sufferer to understand.

4. Do not assume that the person remembers; he or she is likely not to, even though what you refer to may be a daily event.

5. Try to give additional facial and gestural clues to assist understanding.

Mental illness

Mental functioning can be changed by physical diseases for which the cause is known, such as viruses or tumours that affect the brain. Other conditions which have unknown causes, such as depression, psychosis and neurosis, may affect the main areas of mental functioning, which are:

• **mood** which may be angry, happy, sad...

• **cognition** which includes the ability to think, remember, understand and learn

• **behaviour** which includes the way that we react, the tasks that we perform and the way we carry them out.

Changes in mental functioning can have a profound effect on communication. Much of what the person says may reflect the problems they are having in thinking and behaving normally. In other cases, such as severe depression, the person may rarely communicate or even become totally mute. Occasionally people suffering from mental illness can be verbally and physically abusive (see pages 25-26). It is important to try to find out about an individual with a mental illness, and the best way to approach them (see also Chapter 17).

Here are some general guidelines:

• approach the person slowly in a calm and gentle manner

• speak normally but allow them time to understand

• give the person lots of reassurance

• try to gain the person's trust before carrying out any procedures with them

• always explain what you need to do and why

• show the person any equipment you are going to use, and allow them time to ask questions

• try to remember that the person may feel bewildered or frightened and this may show itself as aggression or lack of co-operation.

Learning disabilities

People with learning disabilities (see Chapter 18) may grow physically at a normal rate, but their mental functioning, and sometimes their emotional functioning too, is delayed. Some people with learning disabilities do not reach the usual adult level of functioning and are sometimes described as having a mental age of five, ten or whatever.

It is important to try to find out more about the person from the staff with whom you work or from the person's friends or relatives. However general guidelines to assist communication are as follows:

• approach the person as an adult, if they are so in age

• speak in a normal voice but give one piece of information at a time and allow time for the person to take in the information

• if the person is having difficulty in understanding, cut out all unnecessary detail and concentrate on conveying the important information

• give them plenty of reassurance and try to get to know them

• observe carefully the things that they seem to cope with and the things that they find difficult, so that you can try to speak to the person at the right level for their understanding

• the person may have difficulty in learning and remembering, so that they may need repetitions and frequent reminders.

Children in hospital

Probably the most important point when talking to children in hospital is to have realistic expectations of what they can understand at their age. Most children begin to use words to ask for things at about two years of age, but you need to think about the way you speak to any child under five. (See Chapter 19.)

Just as parents will often make up games to help children eat or behave reasonably in the car on a long journey, the same kind of games can be used with children in hospital to help at mealtimes and in carrying out routine care procedures.

By the age of five most children who are developing normally have a good grasp of language, speak clearly and have a large vocabulary. They can understand most of what is said to them but some aspects of language such as jokes and sarcasm are still too difficult for them. You can still hear immaturities in their speech, but the basic language system is working well and you should be able to understand them easily.

Some children do not develop speech and language for a number of reasons such as hearing deficits, learning difficulties (mental handicap), emotional difficulties, physical handicap and prolonged illness. When working with children in hospital, it is likely that you will find that some children do have communication problems.

Listen to what the child can say and try to reply at that level. If you are speaking to a five year old child who says "want dolly", which is characteristic of language used by two to three year olds, then you may need to use simpler language when you are talking to them than you would normally use with a five year old.

Some children with physical handicaps such as cerebral palsy may not be able to speak at all but may have developed good understanding of language. Whenever you are unsure, ask the child's parents what their child can understand.

Some children find hospital very frightening and may not want to talk at all. Don't press the child to give you an answer but talk to them reassuringly. If the child's parents are not with the child, tell them that the child is being very quiet and obviously needs reassurance. But remember that even noisy children can be anxious.

Above all, remember that you probably already know how best to talk to a frightened or worried child. Most people who have children of their own, or young relatives, develop their own strategies which work very well!

Below is a list of medical problems that are likely to cause communication problems or disorder in children:

Hearing loss: Some children who are deaf from birth hear very little while other children develop ear infections which usually cause temporary hearing problems.

Head injury due to road traffic accidents, brain tumours, stroke: Head injury in children is unfortunately relatively common; strokes in children are rare but do happen. Any damage to the brain may cause temporary communication problems, but some children may have more long term speech and language problems.

Cerebral palsy and muscle diseases may cause difficulty in using the speech muscles and in producing intelligible speech. Feeding may also be affected.

Cleft lip and palate: children born with clefts of the lip and/or palate are likely to have feeding problems as babies. Usually operations to repair the lip and palate are carried out before the child is one year old, but some children need a succession of operations. These children are prone to problems with speech and may have hearing problems due to repeated ear infections.

Hearing problems

Do not shout at someone who has hearing problems. When you shout or even raise your voice, you distort the normal patterns of speech and make it more difficult for the person to hear you. If the person is a lip reader, shouting will distort your facial movements too.

> **Speaking to a person with hearing difficulty:**
> • **face the person**
> • **speak clearly, do not shout**
> • **repeat exactly what you said if they look puzzled, so that your lip movements are also repeated**

Hospitals are often noisy places in which sound reverberates, and on open wards, particularly with high ceilings, there is almost an echo effect sometimes. Normal ward noises make it much more difficult for the person with a hearing loss to hear, even if they wear a hearing aid.

Hearing aids

When a person uses a hearing aid it is important to check regularly that it is in full working order, and to ensure that it is **switched on** when needed. Models and types of hearing aids vary, but the following points are important:
• **Batteries**. These last between one and three months. When they run out they should be kept, and returned to the issuing audiology department where they can be exchanged for new ones free of charge.

If the aid whistles when switched on, and with the volume turned up, the battery is charged. If you cannot get a whistle, it is dead. Batteries should be checked every week and every day if the person is confused.

• **Volume**. To find the best volume setting, adjust the volume to the point just below where a whistle is heard. Check the whistle does not return if the person shakes their head. Observe the person to see if they seem comfortable with this volume.

• **Plastic tube**. The sound passes through this tube, so it must be kept clean, free of wax and flexible. It should be renewed regularly at the audiology clinic.

• **Ear mould**. This is made for the individual, and cannot be worn by anyone else. The small hole at the end is where the sound enters the ear. If this becomes blocked with wax, the aid is much less efficient.

It is therefore essential that the person's ears are checked for wax every six months. Care staff should check and remove any wax obvious in the *outer* ear every day.

You may find that drawing the curtains round a bed helps to dampen the noise, but you may need to use a quiet day room or office nearby if you are giving the person important information and want to make sure they have heard. Sometimes it may be necessary to write your message down.

Before you talk to someone who has a hearing loss, do switch off any nearby radios or TV.

On some wards for elderly people you may find a very useful communication aid consisting of a microphone, into which you speak, connected to an amplifier which the patient holds to their better ear. This type of hearing aid is sometimes more useful than a conventional hearing aid because it does not pick up the same amount of background noise.

Communication aids

Both adults and children who have long term communication problems may have a communication aid. Sometimes the aid is a portable computer or a similar electronic device which has a screen and some form of print-out. When you have spoken to the person, give them time to use the communication aid and look at the screen for their answer. Remember to speak to the person and not the screen!

Speech and language therapy

Speech and language therapists (formerly called speech therapists) provide a service to people with communication impairments or swallowing disorders. Anyone who has difficulty understanding, whose speech is not clear, or who has reading or writing problems may benefit from this service. Most large hospitals have a department to whom patients may be referred. Speech and language therapists will assess someone referred to them, give advice to staff, other carers and family and, where appropriate and possible, they will treat the problem.

Sometimes people are not referred for therapy if they have no speech, but speech and language therapists also help the speechless, sometimes by providing a communication aid for the patient. On the other hand, sometimes after a stroke, a patient may be speaking quite well but have difficulties reading or writing which the therapist may also be able to help.

If you think someone has a communication problem or swallowing disorder, you can ask for them to be referred to your local department.

Points to remember

Being a good communicator involves much more than just hearing accurately and speaking clearly. It involves establishing a rapport with the person by making them feel that you are really listening. So:

1. Establish appropriate posture and position, such as facing someone and perhaps sitting or kneeling to be at their level.
2. Look at the person and establish eye contact.
3. Show that you are interested by listening carefully, nodding appropriately, and responding to what the person says.
4. Use a gesture such as touching their arm for reassurance, where appropriate.
5. Speak in a way that makes the person feel that what they want or are asking about is considered important.
6. Encourage people to talk about themselves, but also about more neutral topics such as the weather, or what has been happening on the news, or in their family.
7. Maintain politeness and do not invade a person's privacy. Remember that people may have different views from you on what is an appropriate topic for conversation.

NVQ Levels 2 & 3 Value Base Units

Oc Promote and support individual rights and choice within service delivery.
Od Acknowledge individuals' personal beliefs and identity.
Oe Support individuals through effective communication.

Levels 2 & 3 Core Units

U5 Obtain, transmit and store information relating to the delivery of a care service.
Z1 Contribute to the protection of indivduals from abuse.

Level 3 Core Units

Z4 Promote communication where there are communication difficulties.

CHAPTER 4

Helping visually handicapped people

Rose Ashbee

- *How to help and communicate with blind and partially sighted people*
- *Sign languages • Guiding, and safety in the environment*

Adapting to change is hard for most of us, but blind and partially sighted people have special difficulties. There are many ways we can help them adjust to an unfamiliar environment; most important is the way we communicate with them.

Communication

When you approach a visually handicapped person, always introduce yourself, say who you are and what your job is. Do stop and chat if you have the time, and always say what you are doing. Try and remember to address each individual by name – after all, they cannot see that you are talking to them. Never leave without saying goodbye: it is frustrating and embarrassing for a person to realise that they are talking to an empty space. Do not shout: many visually handicapped people have excellent hearing. Speak clearly and at a normal pitch.

How easily someone who is deaf and blind can communicate depends on several factors. Firstly, how old they were when they lost their sight and hearing, secondly whether they lost both senses at once or one after another and thirdly whether they have learned a language beforehand, either speech or sign.

Language and speech are not the same thing. Language is the ability to understand and communicate information. Speech is one method of doing this, gesture and touch are others.

People whose first handicap was deafness may know British sign language and finger spelling. They should not find it too difficult to use the deaf blind manual alphabet, as it is an adaptation of the deaf manual spelled out on the hand. An alternative is the Spartan alphabet, block capitals printed on the hand.

If the individual has enough sight you may try using a thick, black felt tipped pen and writing (on paper) in large print. Whatever method you choose, you must use it consistently. It is best to start off by linking it to essential information about some activity, such as meals, dressing or bathing.

Let them touch

When you approach someone who is deaf and blind let them know you are there without startling them, by tapping them gently on the forearm or wrist. To make sure they know who you are, let them feel a ring or a badge or a hair slide that you always wear. Or make an agreed movement on their hand such as tickling their palm gently.

Don't be put off if a deaf and blind person wants to use touch; remember it is the most important information sense they have left. Do use every opportunity to communicate and involve them in what is going on around them.

Guiding

Do ask first if a person wants assistance: no one likes to be grabbed and dragged. Let the person take your arm and walk slightly in front of them, watching out carefully for obstacles. If you need to walk in single file, through an open doorway for example, indicate this by tucking your guiding hand behind your back.

Always stop at the beginning of stairs and steps and say whether they are going up or down and about how many there are. If there is a handrail put the person's hand on it to help them. Make sure you say when you have reached the last step.

Help the visually handicapped person to sit down by putting their hand on the back of the chair. Leave the rest to them; never lower them bodily into a chair they have not inspected.

Mealtimes

Always ask what an individual likes and dislikes. There is nothing worse than putting an item of food into your mouth that you dislike. When serving a meal do remember to say that you have done so. Say what it is and the position it occupies on the plate and stick to the same system. For example, always place meat at 12 o'clock, potatoes at 6 o'clock and vegetables at 3 and 9 o'clock (see page 46 in Chapter 6, Eating and drinking).

Do ask if help is needed, perhaps by cutting up the food. Providing a plate with an upturned rim will assist the visually handicapped person to feed themselves and reduce the risk and embarrassment of food sliding onto the table. When serving drinks say where you are placing them, and never over-fill cups or glasses; this will reduce the risk of spillage.

Dressing

Just because a person cannot see how they look does not mean to say that they do not want to look nice. Never let a visually handicapped person go about with odd coloured shoes on, laddered stockings, untidy hair or grubby clothing. They will rely on you to tell them tactfully if anything is amiss.

The environment

Make sure that the visually handicapped person knows the position of the call system, the radio, bedside locker and shaving points. Even people registered as blind may have some degree of sight. This does not mean that they are able to "see", but they may perhaps be able to distinguish between light and dark. Visual handicaps are so variable and the conditions that enable people to make the best use of their eyesight may vary considerably. Make sure the individual knows where the light switches are.

Make sure they know how to get to the bathroom, lavatory, day room and dining area. Try to mention easy to touch landmarks, such as pictures on the wall, or a change in surface from carpet to tiling underfoot. Watch out for hazards in their path such as hoovers, commodes, trailing flexes or tea trolleys. Always say if you have to leave something in the way, or if something must not be touched. If you move anything always put it back exactly in the same place.

Never put a visually handicapped person's belongings away before asking where they should go.

A little extra help

Do not worry about saying things like "Do you see what I mean?". Avoiding using such terms can often create more difficulties for everyone if a silence follows while you search for a different word.

Be natural. Your tone of voice and your manner is vitally important; it must convey what you intend it to. Visually handicapped people cannot see your face, whether you are smiling, worried or cross. Do not be afraid to touch. A friendly pat on the back or a squeeze of the hand can be reassuring and comforting.

But the greatest need for most deaf or blind people is for companionship. Someone to talk to them at their own pace. To tell them what is going on in the world outside as well as in the hospital. Remember that visually handicapped people are normal people who just can't see. Treat them as you would treat anyone else, except at those times when they need a little extra help. Just as you would in their place.

Points to remember

1. Address each individual by name and always introduce yourself. Stop and chat if you have time, and never leave without saying goodbye.

2. Don't be put off if a deaf and blind person wants to use touch.
3. Ask if someone wants assistance – never grab and drag.
4. At mealtimes, special help will be needed.
5. Don't let people go about looking grubby or untidy.
6. Make sure they know how to get to the bathroom, lavatory, day room and dining area.
7. Watch out for hazards and tell blind people about them.
8. Remember that their greatest need is for companionship.

Resources
National Deaf Blind Helpers League, 18 Rainbow Court, Paston Ridings, Peterborough PE4 6UP. Tel: 0733 73511. Information, advice and publications, including illustrated instructions for manual alphabets. .
Royal National Institute for the Blind, 224 Great Portland St, London W1N 6AA. Advice, information and publications, especially Braille books, periodicals and music, and Moon books and periodicals.

NVQ Levels 2 & 3 Value Base Units
Oc Promote and support individual rights and choice within service delivery.
Oe Support individuals through effective communication.

Level 3 Core Unit
Z4 Promote communication where there are communication difficulties.

Level 2 Direct Care Endorsement
Z10 Enable clients to eat and drink.
Z9 Enable clients to maintain their personal hygiene and appearance.

CHAPTER 5

Personal hygiene and dressing

John Swiatczak

• Different people, different needs • Nursing care plans – helping you to give individual care • Bathing in bed • Help with washing • Care of mouth, eyes, nails, hair, and shaving • Dressing • Choosing and caring for clothes • Special care for people with prostheses • Staff hygiene – preventing cross infection

Washing and dressing are practical skills, learned in childhood, which normally remain with us throughout our adult lives. There are, however, occasions when circumstances change and individuals require assistance. The care assistant plays an important role in helping patients to perform these essential activities of living.

This chapter will look at both practical and psychological needs of patients during what may be a stressful time for a normally independent and active person. The amount of help each patient requires will vary, according not only to the area in which you work, but also to the condition, needs and wants of each patient.

Different needs

There are several reasons why patients may need assistance with hygiene and dressing. One of the most obvious is if the patient is a baby or young child. Here your role may be assisting the parent rather than giving direct care to the patient. This help may include providing the appropriate facilities and equipment or giving parents support and advice if they are unsure of how to deal with an ill child or one with a wound.

A patient who has undergone surgery may depend on the care assistant for their hygiene needs for a short period of recovery after the operation. This is an assisting phase where the patient does not need to re-learn the skills but needs to recover physically in order to undertake them.

In medical areas, patients may be admitted following a heart attack. In this case each consultant will have their own regime that says how much or little individual patients can undertake during their recovery period. Each patient will recover at a different rate and therefore may undertake care of their own hygiene at different times.

On orthopaedic areas patients are often immobilised for long periods and are unable to attend to their own needs in the same way as normal. While they require assistance, remember that they need to learn adaptive skills such as washing in bed rather than in the bathroom. These patients will of course resume their usual activities following recovery.

In areas for care of elderly people there are often patients who have to re-learn or adapt substantially their normal hygiene practices. One reason may be a condition such as cerebro-vascular accident (stroke) which can disable the patient permanently.

Another reason may be chronic ill health, related to arthritis, heart/chest conditions, poor vision or hearing. These patients may require a great deal of direct care, but at the same time the care assistant may be involved in helping the patient to learn to do as much as possible for themselves.

Nursing care plan

In whichever specialty you work, you will work with and under the guidance of a qualified nurse. The qualified nurse responsible for the care of the individual patient will have assessed and planned, in conjunction with the patient, a nursing care plan. This is an individual guide to the nursing care required for that patient.

The care plan usually covers all activities of living including hygiene and dressing and will give an accurate record of all care which has been given. This should be followed consistently and it is important that before beginning any care for the patient the care plan is read and its instructions carefully followed.

It is the role of the qualified nurse to plan care and the role of the care assistant to carry out areas of that care plan with appropriate supervision unless there is a marked change in the patient's condition. In this case the care assistant

must report back to the nurse in charge of the patient's care, before starting any care task.

Principles into practice
Giving assistance with hygiene and dressing requires many practical skills. Each hospital/unit will have its own policies and procedures, but there are basic general principles which should be followed. Most important of all is to remember to take note of each individual patient's needs and preferences.

Bathing in bed

The following is an example of the basic principles to be followed when washing/bathing a patient in bed:

• It is important before commencing any delivery of care that both the patient and member of staff concerned are fully prepared. For a bed bath the patient should be asked if they wish to bathe and the basic procedure should be explained to them. If the patient has any objections these should be noted and acted upon accordingly. This may mean for example that patients are bathed by relatives, or that they do not bathe while in hospital but attend to their own needs as far as possible.

• It is usual for two members of staff to bathe a patient in bed, particularly if the patient is very ill or disabled. Two people are needed to position the patient and to assist with any movements needed during the bath.

• The care assistant will usually be assisting a qualified nurse or learner nurse and the care plan must be read before you start.

• Staff must be aware of embarrassment and stress which may be caused during bathing. If the patient wishes to be bathed by a member of the same sex this should be arranged wherever possible.

• The room or cubicle in which the patient is being nursed should be warm and free from draughts. Any curtains should be drawn, doors closed and screens used as required.

• All the items patient and staff need should be available close to hand. The usual items will be: hot and cold water, soap, flannels, towels, sheets, toiletries, nightwear or other clothing, shaving equipment (if appropriate), toothpaste and brush, linen skip and waste bags.

• The patient must be as involved as possible and should attend to their own needs as far as their condition allows.

• Staff must remember to ask the patient at every stage what they would like. Some people use soap, others don't, some use deodorant, talc etc. Never assume that you know what the patient needs or wants.

• Always dry skin thoroughly, taking particular care around areas where skin surfaces are in contact with each other, such as the groin, below breasts and under arms, as chafing and soreness can occur. This is also an ideal time to observe the patient's skin condition, and the care assistant should be looking for any bruising, redness, sores, oedema (swelling) or rashes, which must then be reported to the nurse responsible for the patient's care. Take great care drying betwee an elderly person's toes, as the skin can easily be damaged.

• Throughout the bed bath it is important to expose the patient as little as possible and also to talk *to* the patient and not *over* them. This is an opportunity to chat, give information and reassure the patient.

Care and independence

The principles relating to bed bathing also relate to assisting with washing in the bathroom or by the bedside, when only one member of staff may be needed. Staff must always remember not to do for a patient anything they can do for themselves, as this can create dependence.

There are several other areas which are part of hygiene care:

Mouth care

Patients who have their own teeth must have access to brushes, paste, mouthwash etc as required. If dentures are worn you may need to clean them for the patient. Use the patient's own preferred cleaning items, and ensure that facilities are available for patients to care for their own dentures if possible. Patients with specific mouth problems will have care planned for them which will be set out in their care plan.

Eye care

Some patients may require eye care – for example patients who are unconscious. This will be set out in the care plan and must be carried out as planned.

Nail care

Nails must be checked regularly and should be kept clean. Nails which are sharp or too long should be cut as required. Care assistants should also know when to refer patients to the qualified nurse for chiropody services, for example if there is any infection present, or if nails are particularly long or difficult to cut.

Hair care

Hair must be kept clean and should be brushed or combed to the patient's liking. They should do it themself

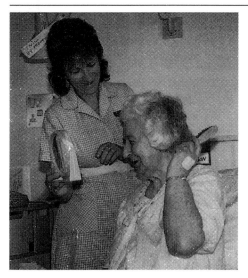

Always encourage patients to do as much as possible for themselves.

wherever possible, but you will need to help by providing and positioning a mirror and making sure they have everything they need. Hair can be washed even if the patient is in bed as bedheads can easily be removed. Most hospitals also offer hairdressing facilities to patients.

Shaving

Facilities must be provided for this. If the patient requires assistance the care assistant should use the patient's own equipment if available. It is important to remember to use clean, sharp razors to reduce skin trauma. If using an electric shaver, it should be checked and cleaned before and after use. Razors must never be shared, because of the risk of cross infection.

Some patients need you to do everything for them (but remember to ask how they would like things done). Others only need help with shaving, for example, or washing their back. Care assistants must ensure that they only give the amount of care the patient requires.

Dressing

Some patients in hospital will not be in bed wearing nightwear but will be encouraged to dress during the day. This is particularly common in paediatric, elderly, mental health and learning disability areas. Although most patients will have no problems with dressing there may be others who require assistance. This can range from help with buttons to learning how to dress completely.

Patients who experience difficulty with dressing may have been referred to the occupational therapist and/or the physiotherapist, both of whom are important members of the multi-disciplinary team. The patient will be assessed by the occupational therapist and the physiotherapist and areas of need plus aids and adaptations will be identified. These may include simple aids such as shoe horns or velcro fastenings or major aids such as wheelchairs or bathroom adaptations.

If appropriate the patient's relative or carer will be encouraged to participate in their care. This is particularly important if the patient has a permanent disability and will need assistance on discharge. The care assistant should work closely with the patient and carer and may act as a link person ensuring that all who will assist the patient carry out that care in the same way.

Patients undergoing a dressing programme must be allowed to do as much as possible for themselves. It is often easier for the care assistant to do something for a patient, particularly if they are having difficulty or are taking a long time. However this can create greater dependence and slow down the rehabilitation process.

The dressing programme will be written down and must be adhered to at all times by all staff to maintain continuity. Any aids or adaptations required by the patient must be kept available at all times. Although it is not possible for the care assistant to know every aid, they should be familiar with those used by the patients in their care.

Dressing programmes can be very frustrating and tiring for the patient and it is vital that the care assistant is always supportive and reassuring.

After surgery

Dressing may be difficult for patients who have wounds or intravenous infusions. The care assistant can help the patient to adapt to the situation by teaching simple things such as how to put on a sleeve over an intravenous site. Patients may need a lot of reassurance, support and encouragement.

Caring for clothes

It is also part of the care assistant's role to care for patients' clothing while in hospital. Many hospitals have facilities where patients' clothing can be laundered. If so it is vitally important that the clothing is labelled clearly and correctly and returned to the right patient.

If patients have to use clothing which belongs to the hospital, please only give them clothes which fit! The days when patients spent the day in ill-fitting and badly laundered clothes should be long gone. **Always** ask the patient what they would like to wear, and as far as possible encourage them to choose their own clothing.

Prostheses

A prosthesis is an artificial part of the body, such as a false limb. Patients with prostheses may need extra psychological as well as practical support. It is possible that no one other than partner/carer has seen the patient without the false leg or eye.

It may be that the patient has been admitted to hospital for surgery after which a prosthesis will be needed, and care assistants will need to assist with dressing until the patient is rehabilitated fully. You must be aware of and able to control your own reactions and facial expressions, as these can cause distress to the patient. Staff must strive to be as calm and supportive as possible.

If a prosthesis appears to be ill-fitting or is causing pain or discomfort to the patient, this must be reported immediately. The care assistant will help the patient to learn new techniques for dressing which will be planned by the multi-disciplinary team.

Staff hygiene

There are several points to remember when discussing hygiene, which are relevant to staff. The risk of cross infection (transferring infection from one person to another) is increased in hospital where several patients with infections are together in a small area, cared for by a small number of staff.

Each hospital will have its own procedures and policies regarding cross-infection, but there are several principles which should be followed:

• Uniform should not be worn outside the workplace, and this includes travelling to and from the hospital.

• Aprons must be worn for any dirty procedure such as bathing or toileting patients. A clean apron must also be worn for clean procedures such as giving out food or carrying out dressings. It is important that staff put on a fresh apron for each procedure.

• Gloves should be worn when dealing with body substances such as blood, urine, faeces, saliva, sputum and vomit, and discarded after each procedure.

• Hand washing must be carried out thoroughly – between fingers, backs of hands and wrists. Washing should continue for at least one minute with soap; hands must then be rinsed thoroughly and dried. Handwashing is particularly important after carrying out any dirty procedure, and before and after serving food. Always wash your hands when you have carried out care for one patient **before** you move on to another.

Body odour

One other aspect of hygiene is body odour. This can be particularly offensive to patients who are in hospital and feel ill. During a busy shift on a warm ward area everyone will sweat; it is therefore important that all staff wash areas such as underarms regularly, and that clean uniform is worn each day. Antiperspirants and deodorants are a personal choice, however sweat does not smell unless it is allowed to become stale on the skin surface or on clothing which is then worn again.

Points to remember

1. The care assistant should always be supportive, encouraging and reassuring.
2. Each patient is an individual with their own needs and preferences.
3. Always read the patient's care plan before delivering care.
4. Always ask. Never assume you know best.
5. Remember that patients can suffer distress and embarrassment through lack of thought.
6. Never create dependence by doing things for the patient which they can do for themselves.

NVQ Levels 2 & 3 Value Base Units
Oc Promote and support individual rights and choice within service delivery.
Oe Support individuals through effective communication.

Levels 2 & 3 Core Units
U4 Contribute to the health, safety and security of individuals and their care environment.
U5 Obtain, transmit and store information relating to the delivery of a care service.

Level 2 Direct Care Endorsement
Z9 Enable clients to maintain their personal hygiene and appearance.
Z6 Enable clients to maintain and improve their mobility.

CHAPTER 6

Helping patients to eat and drink

Wendy Hewitt-Sayer and Ally Lallmahomed

• When people are ill they need more food, not less, but they may have little appetite • What is a balanced diet? • Food supplements and tube feeding • The effects of inadequate nutrition • Choice of meals, including special diets • How to present food, prepare patients for meals, and help them afterwards • The art of feeding patients • Aids to eating • Observing, reporting and recording • Principles of food handling

The amount of food a person needs to meet their body's daily requirements varies according to their age, sex, size, amount of activity, the nature of their work and the climate. Generally bigger, younger, active adults in colder conditions need more food. But ill-health or injury also increases the body's need for nutrition, at a time when people may have a reduced appetite or a physical condition that makes eating or digestion difficult.

Nutrition is a very important factor in a patient's overall care. Without appropriate diet (food and fluid) and sufficient nourishment, treatment programmes will be less effective and the recovery of the patient delayed. The care of the patient at mealtimes is therefore vitally important, and care assistants are centrally involved in delivering this care.

Everyone needs a "balanced diet" in order to keep healthy. A balanced diet is one where the intake of food and fluid contains an adequate amount of the different kinds of nutrients required to meet the body's needs whether one is healthy or ill. These nutrients include protein, carbohydrate, fats, vitamins, mineral salts, fibre and water. Proteins, carbohydrates and fats are energy producing food.

Proteins contain the basic building blocks for body tissues, amino acids, which are essential for growth and repair. They are found in lean meat, fish, egg white, cheese, milk, pulses (lentils etc) nuts and cereals. There are different types of amino acid in vegetable, fish and animal protein, so a variety of food is needed to meet the body's needs completely.

Carbohydrates are needed for energy and are found in potatoes, flour, rice, pulses, milk, sugar, honey, fruits and root vegetables. If there is inadequate intake of carbohydrate to meet energy requirements, this will eventually result in wasting of body tissue.

Fats are found in dairy products, eggs, oils, oily fish, margarine, some fruits (nuts and olives) and fat meat.

Vitamins are essential for the normal functioning of the body. There are many types and each has a different function. Vitamins A,B,C,D and K are the most important ones. Sources of vitamins are liver, dairy products, meat, root and green vegetables, vegetable oil, milk, yoghurt, nuts, pulses.

Minerals (found in food as salts or electrolytes) are needed in very small amounts. Sodium, potassium, calcium, iron, magnesium, iodine and zinc are some examples. Sources of minerals are dairy products, fruit, vegetables, cereal products, meat, fish, poultry, pulses and table salt.

Fibre is a special type of carbohydrate which helps prevent constipation and other bowel disorders. Sources of fibres include cereals, wholemeal flour, wholegrain breads, brown rice, beans, peas, lentils and fruits.

Fluid: The amount of fluid required by the body in each 24-hour period is approximately 2.5 litres for an adult of average size. Part of this fluid will be within food eaten; the rest is taken in the form of drinks. Most adults in hospital need to drink at least 1.5 litres a day.

Protein for growth and healing – in meat, fish, eggs, milk, cheese, yoghurt, nuts, beans and lentils, bread.

Carbohydrate for energy – in bread, flour, pasta, rice, cereals, sugar, fruit and vegetables.

Fats – in meat, fish, chicken, milk, cream, butter, oils, biscuits and cakes.

Fibre to prevent constipation and bowel disorders – in fruit, vegetables, wholegrain and oat cereals and baking, wholemeal bread, beans and lentils.

Calcium for strong bones and teeth – in milk, cheese and yoghurt, canned fish, green leafy vegetables, white bread.

Vitamin C to fight infection and aid healing – potatoes, citrus fruit such as oranges, fruit juice, green vegetables, berry fruits.

Some of the important food groups in a balanced diet.

Nutrition and illness

During illness, energy needs increase because of the extra demands made on the body to repair damage or fight illness. Unfortunately, illness may cause people either to lose their appetite, or to experience difficulty in eating, or both.

Loss of appetite may be due to losing the sense of taste, a painful mouth or difficulty in chewing or swallowing. People may not be able to feed themselves easily, they may have pain or be depressed. All these can result in insufficient quantity and quality of food being eaten.

If someone with a swallowing problem is allowed to eat and drink, there is a risk of either choking or food entering the lungs. Once food or fluid is in the lungs, chest infections may be the result. It is therefore vital to follow the correct procedures and to ask if you are at all unsure of what to do.

Food supplements

Patients often have very small appetites and find they cannot manage much food at mealtimes. Small snacks in between meals can help to ensure they take in enough nourishment. Other patients cannot take solid food because of swallowing difficulties. They may need a soft diet to be ordered for them, or food supplements.

There are various food supplements in the form of drinks which provide all the necessary nutrients for the patient. There are various brands of drinks, flavoured sweet or savoury, available on the market. The dietitian will advise which is the most appropriate to meet the patient's needs, taking into account both the patient's preferences and dietary requirements.

Tube feeding

Some patients may require a higher level of technical assistance with feeding due to difficulty in swallowing, diminished level of consciousness or surgery. Patients may also have a nutritional requirement which is greater than their appetite (for example if they have severe burns or other form of large wound).

A fine tube (nasogastric) may be passed through the nasal passage, down the oesophagus and into the patient's stomach. Alternatively a feeding (gastric) tube may be inserted through the abdominal wall into the stomach.

When providing general care to this group of patients, you must ensure that the tubes are not dislodged. It is important to report to a qualified nurse any problems such as the patient's discomfort, disconnection of the tube to the feeding line, irritation around the nostril, or nose bleed. Under no circumstances should the care assistant manipulate the tube, as it could end up positioned in such a way that breathing is affected.

Inadequate nutrition

If a person does not take in enough food and fluids to supply their daily energy and body repair needs, it will eventually lead to physical and mental changes.

The physical symptoms include loss of weight, a general sense of weakness and illness, muscle weakness, delayed healing and reduced resistance to infection. With loss of skin elasticity, and reduction in fat and muscle layers, people will be at greater risk of developing pressure sores.

Mental symptoms include depression, anxiety, irritability, loss of concentration and apathy. Children's growth and mental development will be impaired, perhaps permanently, if there is inadequate nutrition over a long period of time.

Your vital role

It would be difficult to overstate the importance of a patient's diet in maintaining or ensuring a return to physical, mental and social wellbeing. The care assistant has an important role in ensuring that:

• each patient receives the food he/she requires

• food is presented attractively and the portion size is appropriate

• the patient is positioned so that they can reach their food and eat easily

• if the patient needs special "aids" or equipment, these are clean and available on the meal tray or table

• patients are fed by staff where this is necessary

• the patient's food intake is always observed, and is recorded when requested.

Choosing food

Patients should be assisted to choose their own meals from the menu – everyone has their own particular likes and dislikes. Help may be needed if patients have difficulty reading the menu, understanding the menu choices or writing on menu cards, or they may be unfamiliar with the hospital routines and what the patient is expected to do. It is probably true to say that the patients who need the most help are the ones for whom the right choice is most important.

Special diets

It is essential to know whether the patient is on a special diet such as diabetic, reducing, low potassium, low salt or fat free diets. These diets should be recorded by the nurses in the patient's care plan, and usually an information sheet will be provided for the patient by the dietitian.

Cultural needs

An increasing proportion of people do not eat meat. Some of those who do not eat meat may eat fish. Some vegetarians will not eat any form of meat, fish, eggs or dairy produce.

People from ethnic groups such as Hindus, Moslems and Jews have specific rules about food and its preparation. Hindus do not eat meat. Moslems and Orthodox Jews only eat meat from animals slaughtered in specific ways, they do not eat pork or any food which has been prepared with pork.

These are just three, brief examples of the many cultural and religious beliefs of patients. It is important to learn as much as you can about the beliefs and lifestyles of the people you care for; there is a considerable amount of literature on the subject now (see Chapter 11 *Resources*). If there is nothing on the menu that is suitable for the patient to eat, this should be reported to the nurse in charge so that other arrangements can be made.

The right meal

Having taken care to ensure that the patient has chosen a meal which is

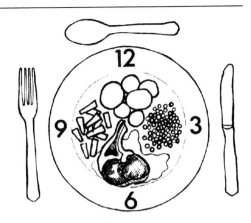

It helps to use the idea of a clock face to describe their plate of food to a blind person.

acceptable to them, don't forget to check at mealtimes that patients actually receive the meal they have chosen!

Presentation of food

Mealtimes are a very important time of day for patients. The care assistant can do a great deal to influence patient's enjoyment of their meals. Presentation of food can have a strong effect on the person's appetite.

Trays, cutlery and crockery should always be spotlessly clean, and attractively presented. Knives, forks, spoons and napkins should be set out tidily, seasoning and condiments to hand.

The food on the plate should be arranged so that the components of the meal are separately identifiable. If there are any drips spilt in the process of serving, these should be wiped off with a clean cloth or paper towel.

If you are giving a meal to a blind or partially sighted person, you will need to tell them how you have organised their food and meal tray. It is customary to describe the placement of food on a plate, using either clock or compass terminology (see diagram above).

The right size of meal

The portions should not be too large as this can be off-putting to someone with a small or absent appetite. Neither should they be too small for someone with a big appetite, or who is particularly hungry.

Preparing for meals

Hospital wards will vary in the dining facilities they offer: some will be homely, others more clinical. Whatever the physical environment, attention should be paid to making mealtimes pleasurable and relaxed. Disturbance and interruption should be avoided so that patients can eat their meal while it is still fresh and/or hot.

Washing hands

Some people like to wash their hands or go to the toilet before their meal, but may not like to ask. The care assistant needs to check with each patient and offer them the chance to wash or visit the toilet if they wish to.

Dentures

Not all patients wear their dentures all day. You must check that dentures are clean, and help to insert the denture if necessary.

Sitting at a table

Whenever possible encourage patients to sit out for their meals or assist them to the dining room. Patients in bed need to be sat upright, if they are able to do so.(If you are unsure how much activity is advisable or possible for a particular patient, always check with a trained nurse.) The bed table should be positioned at a convenient height, cleared of unnecessary items and have the meal tray and a drink within easy reach.

Medicine

Some people may need medication before their meal. A diabetic patient may require tablets or an insulin injection, others may need indigestion medication. Although health care assistants are not responsible for medicines, it is important they are aware of each patient's requirements.

Signs and instructions

Before serving a meal, check the person's care plan for any information on feeding methods and special diets; also their bed for any "Nil by mouth", "Fluids only" or other diet signs used in your ward.

Feeding aids

There are many types of adapted cutlery and utensils to help meet the specific needs of individual patients.

Knives, forks and spoons are made with larger and shaped handles for easier use by someone with a weak grip, for example following a stroke or because of arthritis. There are forks with a cutting edge for people who can only use one hand.

Plate guards can prevent spilling of food and to help push food onto forks or spoons. Sticky mats ensure plates do not move when patients are cutting up food. There are cups with spouts, two handled beakers and drinking straws. These are only some of the many aids available to help patients feed themselves.

Occupational therapists will be able to provide advice where there are particular difficulties. They are trained to assess the patient, and may have access to a wider range of equipment than is generally available on the wards.

Do remember, however, that patients may be sensitive about their disability, and may prefer to use "normal" cutlery. Their views should be respected and assistance given, either without aids or with aids which they find acceptable.

Protection of clothes is also an area where sensitivity is required. If clothes are likely to become soiled in the course of eating, due to spillage etc, this should be anticipated. A range of "bibs", plastic or disposable may be available; these will be welcomed by some patients while others may feel humiliated. A thought in advance could save the patient the indignity of soiling their clothes and the need to change them.

Helping patients eat

The amount of help needed by individuals will vary. Some, if prepared well, will be able to feed themselves. Others will require feeding with their entire meal.

You will know which patients are going to need help. Make sure that the person is sitting up and not tilted back, and those who require help to cut food up are given this assistance promptly, so that their meal does not get cold and unappetising. Check with the patient how small they like their food cut up, as this will vary.

Feeding

There is an art to feeding patients, so that they neither feel rushed nor are left waiting for the next mouthful. As a general rule, do not feed patients from a standing position; present food at the same angle as you would feed yourself. Sit with them in such a way that you can see their face, allow sufficient time for them to chew their food and give them your full attention.

Make it a pause in your day and establish a rapport with your patient, so that you can anticipate when they are ready for the next mouthful. You may find that patients use a nod or other non-verbal indication of their readiness.

Offer a drink at intervals. Some people like to drink during a meal, others don't.

Observe, report, record

As part of your general care, it is important to be aware of any patient who does not eat their meal, or who has difficulty. A patient with improved appetite or eating ability is also worthy of note. Your observations should be reported to the trained nurse responsible for the patient. An alternative choice of meal, food supplements or referral to the dietitian may be indicated.

Charts are sometimes kept of the food and fluid eaten (and offered). These should be written promptly and accurately after each meal.

After meals

Patients will need help after meals too, perhaps to wash hands and face, use a mouthwash or clean their dentures. Toilet facilities should also be offered. Some patients may have dropped food on to their clothes; sensitive assistance to change clothes will be needed.

Patients confined to bed should be settled into a comfortable position, and the bed tidied. Care should be taken to remove any crumbs or particles of food in the bedclothes, as these are both unacceptable in terms of comfort and could cause localised pressure damage to patient's skin. Patients who have been helped out of bed for their meal may wish to return to bed.

Food handling

Everyone dealing with food need to comply with certain standards of cleanliness. These include wearing neat and clean clothes, long hair tied at the back. Finger nails should be clean and hands always washed before dealing with patients' food. If a member of staff has a cut on their hand or finger, it should be covered with a clean waterproof plaster or plastic gloves worn. Staff's fingers should not come into direct contact with food or drinks. In some units it is policy for staff to wear disposable plastic aprons to prevent contamination of food from clothes and protect clothes from becoming soiled.

Conclusion

This chapter has looked at the importance of ensuring patients receive adequate nutrition and the important role of care assistants. Good care at mealtimes will help to ensure that a patient's intake of food and fluid is sufficient to meet their needs, to maintain their health and aid their recovery from ill-health, surgery or injury. As with all other aspects of care, meeting a patient's nutritional needs involves taking into account many different factors – social, environmental, cultural and psychological as well as physical.

Points to remember

1. People need a balanced diet to keep healthy.
2. Energy needs are increased during illness due to the extra demands made on the body.

3. Inadequate nutrition can affect people physically and mentally.
4. Patients need to be given a choice of meals.
5. There are many cultural and social factors which influence an individual's choice of food.
6. The presentation of food is important as it can affect a patient's appetite.
7. There are many types of feeding aids to help meet specific needs of the disabled patient.
8. Care assistants have a very important role in meeting patients' nutritional requirements .

NVQ Levels 2 & 3 Value Base Units
Oa Promote antidiscriminatory practice.
Oc Promote and support individual rights and choice within service delivery.
Od Acknowledge individuals' personal beliefs and identity.
Oe Support individuals through effective communication.

Levels 2 & 3 Core Units
U4 Contribute to the health, safety and security of individuals and their care environment.
U5 Obtain, transmit and store information relating to the delivery of a care service.

Level 2 Direct Care Endorsement
Z10 Enable clients to eat and drink.
Z9 Enable clients to maintain their personal hygiene and appearance.
Z11 Enable clients to access and use toilet facilities.

CHAPTER 7

Lifting and handling patients

Stuart Darby

• How to assess the risk of lifting and handling a patient • How to plan a lift
• Staff training • Methods of lifting • Recording and reporting risk factors

Moving furniture, carrying shopping and picking up children are just some of the everyday activities of lifting and handling that we take for granted. Lifting patients and supporting them to transfer from one position to another is an important part of the work of the care assistant. The danger of taking this type of activity for granted is that we no longer concentrate on what we are doing, and so increase the risks of injuring ourselves, our patients or work colleagues.

Important new regulations* came into force in January 1993. These regulations are designed to ensure that all people involved in manual lifting and handling are aware of these risks and only undertake lifting and handling when it is really necessary, as part of a conscious and planned decision.

The new lifting and handling regulations stress the importance for everyone involved in lifting to receive practical training in their place of work. This training should help you to contribute to assessing the risks involved in lifting and handling patients and to take account of your own abilities, the abilities of patients to help themselves, the methods and equipment you may use and the surroundings in which you lift and handle. The regulations stress three main points:

• Lifting and handling should be avoided as far as reasonably practicable.

• Lifting should be planned by a suitably qualified member of staff, and these plans should be recorded and followed.

• Any identified risks or unsafe practices are reported and recorded to prevent accidents or injury as a result of lifting and handling.

Assessing the risk

Before starting any lifting or handling procedure, the risks to both the patient being lifted and the person undertaking the lift must be assessed so that steps can be taken to reduce any threat of injury. The key factors in assessment are:

1. The lifter's ability, knowledge, and fitness to lift.

2. The ability of the person being lifted to assist themselves.

3. The lifting and handling task to be undertaken.

49

4. The surroundings in which lifting and handling will take place.

5. Recording the lifting and handling method.

6. Steps to reduce or remove the risk of injury.

7. Lifting and handling methods.

These key factors are considered in detail in this chapter.

1 The lifter's ability, knowledge, and fitness to lift.

Training and education
Any person required to lift and handle must be offered the opportunity to participate in training and education tailored to their individual needs and the place in which they work.

Training should be provided by qualified practitioners and should aim to provide you with instruction, experience and a knowledge of:
• The Health & Safety at Work Act 1974 and the legal aspects of lifting and handling.
• How the body works in relation to movement and lifting and handling.
• How to assess any risks of injury and report to managers
• How to plan the most appropriate methods for safer patient handling.
• Manual handling techniques and the use of equipment.
• Warning of unsafe handling practice.

Fitness to do the job
It is also important to ensure that as a lifter you are fit to undertake these duties. If you are not fit, you are at risk of back injury because of the strenuous nature of the job. Good health can contribute to your ability to make a reasoned assessment and your proficiency in undertaking the lift.

More than a quarter of accidents at work reported each year are associated with manual handling. The majority result in injuries lasting over three days and occur because of prolonged lifting over a period of time rather than as a result of single accidents. These injuries can result in long term physical problems or even permanent disability.

Appropriate clothing and footwear
Uniforms should be designed to take into account the movements that you will need to make. They must allow you to bend and stretch freely. Where no uniform is worn, it is important that you select clothing that allows free movement, but is unlikely to be caught in equipment. Footwear, in particular rubber soled shoes, will protect you from static electricity and are non-slip on wet or polished surfaces. The upper surface is equally important to protect feet from articles or objects that may be dropped on them.

2 The ability of the person to assist themselves

Promoting independence
Apart from reducing the risk of injury to lifters, promoting independence is important because it allows each person the opportunity to assist and control everyday tasks, to do what they want to, when they need to. It allows each person to have a sense of dignity and fulfilment in carrying out movement and daily living activities without interference and intrusion.

There are however a number of physical and psychological factors that need to be considered in assessment that will prevent or limit the extent to which some patients can assist themselves in lifting and handling. In order to plan the best approach you should also refer to other chapters in this book.

Factors affecting patients' ability to assist with lifting and handling include:

Physical factors.
• The weight, height and shape of the person.
• Normal "wear and tear" to the body, or the process of an illness or disease.
• Decreased elasticity of muscles and the inability to bend and flex easily.
• A decline in strength of bones through bone loss.
• Reduced lung expansion causing breathlessness on effort.
• Poor eyesight and inability to recognise objects, steps or floor changes increases the risk of falls and accidents.
• Changes in the inner ear may cause loss of balance control.
• Medicines and alcohol causing drowsiness and unsteadiness.
• Heart changes, causing blood pressure to rise or fall quickly, may make the person dizzy or unsteady.
• Pain in the hands or limbs, caused through rheumatism or arthritis, can limit a full range of movement.
• The effects of tiredness.
• Other physical constraints (drips, tubes, splints, traction).

Psychological factors
• The ability to remember and recall information or to recognise places or objects, where they are (the time, month or year), and what is happening to them.
• The ability to communicate, speak or to understand what is being said.
• The ability to behave appropriately, including aggression due to frustration, confusion, anxiety or suspicion of any actions carried out.
• "Clinging", which can occur where the person has experienced a fall, feels insecure and has lost self confidence.
• Understanding of the situation (which may be impaired where there has been damage or disease of the brain).
• The mood of the person (happy and relaxed or sad and anxious) may affect their ability to concentrate, or their willingness and motivation to participate.

3 The lifting and handling task to be undertaken

Do I need to lift and handle?
The first question before any lifting task is whether it actually needs to be undertaken, or whether the person can move themselves.

Where lifting or assistance is needed, the point at which the lift will start from and where it will end needs to be clarified. If you are required to twist, stretch or bend in order to carry out the task there is an added risk of injury. The length of time that the lift takes will add to the risk of injury, particularly if it is to be repeated on several occasions during the day. The plan for repeated and regular lifting therefore, needs to ensure that the least stress is placed upon the person and the lifters.

What method should be used?
The type of lifting carried out will depend upon the assessment and characteristics of the person to be lifted, your own abilities, the environment in which you will lift and handle and the range of equipment and staff available to help you.

Preparation for the type of lift to be carried out
The following checklist is a guide to selecting which method of lift to use:
• Can this lift be undertaken manually or does equipment need to be used ?
• Is it a horizontal transfer lift? Can a sliding action be used?
• Does the lift involve pivoting or turning?
• Is it a vertical lift? How much weight has to be lifted?
• Does it involve turning the person in bed?

• What level of support does the person need?

• Is there an additional task to be done, eg changing clothes or using a bedpan?

• Will you be able to maintain a good posture, keeping your body symmetrical and your back straight?

• Do you need more staff to help?

• What equipment may be needed?

Hoists

Hoists may be used for lifting patients in or out of bed, for lifting a person up the bed, raising a person while the lower sheets are changed or the person is being washed, and for lifting patients in the bath and from the floor.

Hoists may be fixed in a certain place, such as bathrooms or they may be mobile. If they are mobile it is essential that you always remember to apply the brakes. Hoists also have many attachments such as seat fittings and slings. You should always use the correct fitting. Remember that there are always manufacturers' representatives who will advise and can even have specially adapted slings made.

Handling or transfer equipment

Equipment is designed to be used as an aid to lifters. Handling and transfer equipment is also designed to be used by patients who can assist themselves and so increase their level of independence after being taught how to use it safely. Practical examples are included in *Lifting and handling methods* below.

All equipment needs to be selected with care, regularly inspected for wear and tear and regularly maintained. If it is available it should always be used. Advice on equipment can be sought from qualified nursing staff, physiotherapists, occupational therapists, or the manufacturers of the equipment. Always seek special training in the use of mechanical hoists.

4 The surroundings in which the lift is taking place

Is the area clear ?

Ensure that you have enough space in which to move around, and that the distance you will be travelling is clear of any objects or items of furniture. If you are transferring a person from one place to another, for example bed to chair, ensure that these are at the same level.

Plan your move to take into account the number of different stages, standing, turning, sitting and so on. Lower any handrails or chair sides to minimise the amount of lifting and lowering required. Be sure to lock the wheels of equipment, and position, for example, a chair or bed ladder which may help the patient to help themselves.

If you are involved in lifting at night, make sure that the area is well lit and that you can see where you are going.

Is the floor safe?

There may be obstacles, such as furniture or rugs and carpets. The floor may be wet, polished or may be covered in talcum powder, or other slippery substances. Do remember that other patients and even pets may be a hazard to look out for.

Clothing and footwear of the person be lifted

It is equally important, where appropriate, for the person being lifted and handled to wear well fitting shoes that support the foot and ankle, and not loose fitting slippers. Remember also that long hair, rings and jewelry can get trapped in clothing and equipment.

5 Recording the lifting and handling method

Care planning

It is good practice for a trained "assessor" to be responsible for making an initial assessment and for documenting care needs in partnership with the patient. A trained assessor is usually a qualified nurse or therapist who has undertaken specialist education in assessing lifting and handling risks and identifying the most appropriate methods and equipment to be used. Assessors are responsible for written care plans and nursing records. Re-assessment should take place whenever required, and following regular review.

Written plans for lifting and handling should include:

• The lift to be carried out.
• How the lift will be carried out.
• The number of lifters required.
• Any environmental considerations or precautions to be taken
• The type of equipment required.
• Agreement that everyone involved, including the person to be lifted, understands the methods to be used and how they might help.

The specific responsibility for each handling task however, lies with each lifter on every occasion that a lift is undertaken. You are responsible for reading and following the care plan. Changes in care should be reported and care plans altered as soon as possible. Where difficulties exist these must be recorded and reported as soon as possible.

6 Steps to reduce or remove the risk of injury

Employer responsibilities

Your employer has a responsibility to ensure that you are fit to lift and handle by providing training, a safe environment and by ensuring that you have the appropriate equipment where available. As an employee you also have a responsibility for the safety of yourself, the patients that you are lifting and handling and the other staff with whom you work. This includes reporting injuries and where there is a lack of resources and equipment.

Injuries, accidents or illness at work

Your manager has a responsibility to ensure that neither the person you are lifting, yourself or your colleagues are exposed to a foreseeable risk of injury from lifting and handling.

Your responsibility is to aim to reduce the risk of injury by reporting and recording where there is a problem or where work place injuries or accidents have occurred. This includes any illness or disability affecting your handling abilities when you are new to post or in the course of your duties, whether relating to a work accident or not. This can be done confidentially through occupational health services and GPs.

Reducing and removing the risk of injury

In order to reduce and remove the chance of injury it is good practice to record and report any risks to your manager. This includes the following:

a) Lack of staff or equipment.
b) Environmental hazards.
c) Defects in machinery or equipment.
d) Injuries or accidents.
e) Any illness or disability affecting your handling ability.

a) Lack of staff or equipment.

• What type of equipment is needed and why?
• Why are more staff required on this occasion?
• Has any previous action been taken?

b) Environmental hazards

• Where does the environmental hazard exist?
• What is the environmental hazard creating difficulty?
• What immediate action can remove or reduce the hazard?

c) Defects in equipment/machinery used for lifting
• What model of equipment is it?
• Has it been maintained recently?
• What is the defect or problem?

d) Injuries or accidents
• When and how did the injury occur?
• What equipment was involved?
• What medical treatment was given or action taken?

e) Any illness or disability affecting your handling ability
• How does this limit your ability to lift and handle?
• Do you need to take any special precautions?
• Do you need any special equipment, or have other requirements?

7 Lifting and handling methods

Holds and lifts
The following limited holds and lifts are intended to illustrate the need for safe and planned lifting and handling. The risks associated with lifting and handling are complex. No responsibility can be accepted for any decisions made solely upon the information in this chapter.

Each individual has a responsibility to ensure that they are trained and competent, are able to assess situations to the best of their abilities and have had the opportunity to participate in demonstrations and controlled practice with a qualified practitioner.

It is essential that explanation of the lift is given to the patient and that the lifter gains cooperation where possible.

HOLDS AND LIFTS: ONE HANDLER
These holds are intended to support and move the person who is able to give some assistance and to bear some of their own weight. They are used to assist a person to stand or transfer from one seated position to another seated position close by – for example from wheelchair to toilet.

For the following holds it is essential that the person is sitting well towards the front of the chair or bed, leaning forward and bringing their centre of gravity over their feet which are well tucked in.

• Handling belt hold (Figure 1)
• The lifting block (Figure 2)
• The turn-table (Figure 3)
• Through arm grasps (Figure 4)

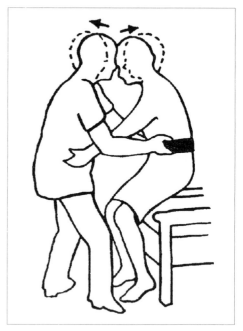

Figure 1: Handling belt hold (above)

1) Stand in front and to one side of the sitting person.

2) Place one foot beside them and the other in front – blocking the person's knees.

3. Insert thumbs in a wide belt (at least three inches) that is secured around the person and grasped. Special belts are available for this purpose.

4. Ask the person to support themselves by pushing up on the arms of a chair or by putting their hands on the lifter's hips.

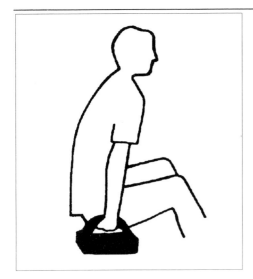

Figure 2: The lifting block (above)

This is useful for patients who may have limited power on one side of the body only.

1) As the lifter lifts, the person pushes down onto the block from a slightly bent elbow on the strong side of the body and pushes onto the strong heel.

2) The lifter adopts the position for the shoulder lift (Figure 8) on the person's weak side but the palm is placed upwards under the person's near thigh, at the same time locking the person's arm if it is paralysed.

Figure 3: The turntable (right)

This may be used for selected patients with caution. It is not suitable for people who are confused or cannot be relied upon to take weight through their knees.

1) Place the person's feet firmly on the turntable and stand to one side of them

2) Hold them with the axillary hold, or belt and keeping close to their body, help them to stand

3) The lifter pushes the turn-table round with their foot until the person is in the correct position to sit on the chair or edge of the bed provided.

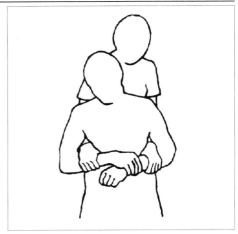

Figure 4: Through arm grasp (above)

1) Hold the person's forearm close to their body. Their stronger hand should grasp the weaker wrist (if appropriate).

2) Stand directly behind them.

3) Grasp as near to their wrist as possible, and tuck their hands into the lower abdomen

This lift is used where the person is seated in an upright position and where they are able to stand, carry some of their own weight, understand and cooperate.

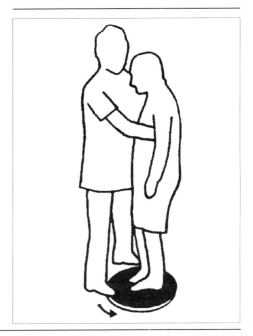

HOLDS AND LIFTS: TWO HANDLERS

Two handlers sharing a lift will still in effect be each bearing two thirds of the total load. The weight may also be unevenly distributed – for example when one lifter has the shoulders and trunk and a second lifter has the feet. At least two lifters should be used where they are manually lifting the whole weight of a person.

- Patient handling sling (Figure 5)
- Double wrist (Figure 6)
- Double forearm (Figure 7)

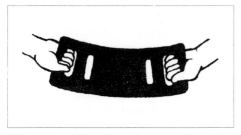

Figure 5: Patient handling sling (above)
The patient handling sling should be used in order to extend the reach and reduce a stooping or twisting action. In the absence of a sling a double wrist hold or a finger hold should be used.

1) The patient handling sling is placed high up under the person's thighs and the lifters hold the sling instead of each others hands.

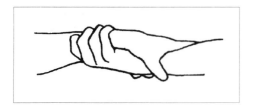

Figure 6: Double wrist hold (above)

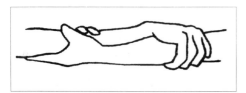

Figure 7: Double forearm hold (above)

Moving patients in bed

- The shoulder lift (Figure 8)
- The through arm lift – up the bed (Figure 9)

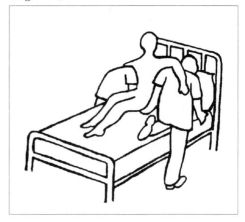

Figure 8: The shoulder lift (above)
Moving in bed or transferring to a chair
1) Adjust the bed to a height halfway between your hips and knees.
2) Apply the brakes
3) Lifters stand on opposite sides to each other with their feet apart.
4) The leading foot should face the moving direction.
5) The hips and knees are bent, with the back straight.
6) Lifters press their near-side shoulders into the chest wall under the person's axilla, while the patient rests their hands and arms down your backs.
7) Grip your partner using the wrist grip.
8) Place your hands on the bed behind the patient to support their trunk, with the elbows flexed ready to take the weight.
9) Leading lifter gives the command "lift".
10) Slowly straighten your trailing legs and elbows.
11) Lift clear of the bed and then lower by bending the leading legs and supporting elbows.
12) Only move the patient for a short distance at a time.

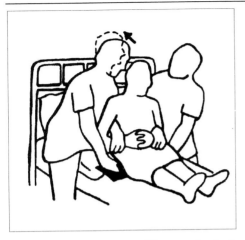

Figure 9: Through arm lift - up the bed or into a chair (above)

1) Put your knee on the bed behind the patient.

2) Using the "through arm grasp", move them to the side of the bed.

3) Place your feet on the floor, behind the client, while continuing to support them.

4) Second lifter positions the chair, then faces the bed with their feet one in front of the other.

5) Second lifter slides their hands under the person's legs.

6) On command, the second lifter pulls the person's legs to the side of the bed, and supports their weight.

7) Lift (using the through arm grasp).

8) Move in this way, for the shortest distance possible, and gently lower to the chair.

Turning the person in bed

Lifting is unnecessary when turning a person in bed. Turning involves rolling and sliding TOWARDS the lifter. This can be achieved in a number of ways.

• Draw sheet or polythene sheet
• Patient handling sling
• Easy-glide boards (Figure 10)

Draw sheet and polythene sheet

A draw sheet or strong sheepskin placed over a polythene sheet to ease gliding can be used to pull the person into position. They should always be supported and comfortable. Care should be take to avoid any friction to the person's skin. No reaching movements should be made away from the lifter, only towards the lifter.

Patient handling slings

Two patient handling slings can be used where there is no draw-sheet. These are positioned under the person's thighs and lower back. Feet, head and shoulders are moved first and then lifters on either side of the bed hold the slings to pull and roll the person's pelvis and trunk.

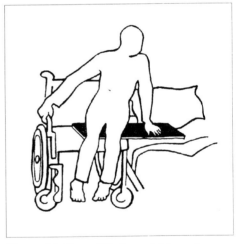

Figure 10: Easy glide board (above)

Easy glide boards are designed to be placed under the person. Specific practical instruction is required to ensure safe use of this equipment.

The falling or fallen patient

Teaching people to fall and rise safely is a skilled activity. Training should be provided by qualified practitioners and should aim to provide the handler and the patient with instructions and practical experience.

Patients who are at risk of falling should be taught firstly, how to fall safely and then how they should rise.

Lifting patients who have fallen to the floor is a very high risk activity. The first task is to ensure that the patient is reassured and made comfortable. Check that they have not sustained any injury. Help should always be summoned and an assessment and well organised lift, preferably using a mechanical hoist, is essential.

Points to remember

1. Each individual has a responsibility to ensure that they are trained, competent, and able to assess situations to the best of their abilities.
2. Never lift a person unless you have to; always consider alternatives.
3. Ensure that everyone involved, including the person you are lifting, knows and understands the plan of lifting and handling: what each person is expected to do, what equipment will be used and any special precautions that need to be taken.
4. Never undertake a lift where the individuals cannot be held close to the body or if your back is twisted.
5. Make certain that there is enough space to lift, it is well lit and that there are no obstacles such as furniture, or hazards such as a slippery floor.
6. Always seek help to move another person unless you are absolutely certain they require minimal support.
7. Never try to stop a person falling –

guide them to the floor.
8. Never lift a person out of the bath or from the floor – use a hoist or bath seat.
9. Never hold the weight of a patient while a nursing activity is being carried out such as wound care or changing clothing or bed linen.
10. Always report to the appropriate manager where there are insufficient staff or equipment, an unsafe environment or faulty equipment with which to lift and handle.

Further reading
*EEC (1990) Minimum Health and Safety requirements for handling loads where there is a risk of back injury for workers. Directive 90/269.EEC.

The Guide to the Handling of Patients 3rd Ed. National Back Pain Association in Collaboration with the Royal College of Nursing (1992).

NVQ Levels 2 & 3 Core Units
U4 Contribute to the health, safety and security of individuals and their care environment.
U5 Obtain, transmit and store information relating to the delivery of a care service.

Level 2 Direct Care Endorsement
Z6 Enable clients to maintain and improve their mobility.
Z7 Contribute to the movement and treatment of clients to maximise their physical comfort.

CHAPTER 8

Pressure area care

Claire Hale

Who is at risk of developing pressure sores • What happens to body tissues under pressure • How to prevent damage • How sores should be treated • Your role

A "pressure sore" is a term used to describe an area of damage to the skin and tissue underneath it, which has been caused primarily by unrelieved pressure. Pressure sores most frequently occur in those patients who cannot move without help.

The most vulnerable group is elderly people, who often sit or lie in the same position for long periods because they are unable to move themselves. This lack of mobility is often caused by some underlying condition such as arthritis, a stroke or a fractured hip following a fall.

However, all patients, including young children, are at risk of developing pressure sores. Nurses who went to Romania found that some of the young physically handicapped children in the orphanages had developed pressure sores because they had been left lying in beds and cots for long periods.

For any patient, young or old, a pressure sore leads to unnecessary suffering, pain and loss of dignity, while nurses and their assistants are likely to develop feelings of guilt, frustration and confusion.

The purpose of this chapter is to provide information about how pressure sores are caused, how they can be prevented, and how they can be treated if they do occur. The final section will look at the role of the care assistant in preventing and treating pressure sores.

The causes of sores

A pressure sore is caused by an interruption to the blood supply to that area. This interruption to the blood supply is usually caused by pressure, of which four types are usually recognised: compression, shearing, direct disruptive damage and friction.

Compression: This occurs when body tissues are squashed between a bone inside the body and a firm surface such as a bed (see diagram 1). The capillaries (tiny blood vessels) lying between the bone and the surface become narrowed or blocked and the blood supply to the tissues reduced. The tissues eventually die from lack of oxygen (which is carried to them in the blood). A patient left sitting too long in one position will suffer from this type of pressure, and a pressure sore will result.

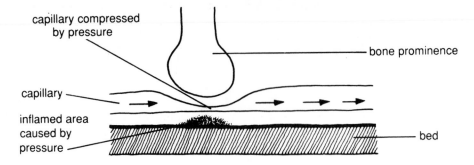

capillary compressed by pressure

bone prominence

capillary

inflamed area caused by pressure

bed

Diagram 1: The effects of compression.

Shearing: Shearing forces are caused by dragging the skin over hard surfaces; the skin's surface becomes grazed and this damages the network of small blood vessels. Patients left in a semi-recumbent position (ie half-sitting, half lying) are liable to this type of damage particularly at their sacrum (the base of the spine) and heels from sliding down the bed (see diagram 2).

Direct disruptive damage: This occurs when a severe blow to the tissues damages the capillaries; this once again causes disruption of the blood supply to the tissues, and tissue death due to lack of oxygen. A patient falling on to a hard surface would be likely to develop this sort of damage.

Friction: This causes burns and abrasions on the skin, and is likely to occur when two areas rub against each other. Sores developing under breasts are one example of this form of pressure. Another kind of "friction sore" is caused by a Plaster of Paris cast rubbing against the skin (also called a **plaster sore**). This occurs when the plaster cast is fitting badly. The patient may complain of a burning sensation inside the plaster. If this occurs the plaster will be removed and re-applied, or else a hole will be cut in the plaster to allow the sore to be dressed.

Knowledge of the different forces that can contribute to pressure sores is important so that they can be avoided. However, not everyone exposed to pressure will go on to develop sores.

A number of additional factors have been identified, which are known to make people more likely to develop sores. These include patient factors such as both increased and decreased body weight, diseases affecting the blood and blood vessels, any kind of reduced mobility, pain and malnutrition. Other factors, which are mainly in the control of ward staff, include poor patient hygiene, poor lifting techniques, hard beds and trolleys and incorrect positioning.

Some patients are generally more likely to get sores than others. These include elderly people, those with spinal injuries causing paralysis and loss of sensation, patients who are sedated or who are taking drugs that are likely to make them sleepy, the terminally ill and any patients with wasting, low resistance to infection, poor nutrition and impaired mobility.

Finally, chairbound people who may seem to be "better off" than bed-bound patients are actually at greater risk of developing sores, because their body weight is not evenly distributed over such a wide area, and because preventive measures may not be applied so rigorously.

To help nurses to identify the patients who are at risk of developing sores, a number of "pressure sore risk calculators" have been developed. These list the factors that make sores more likely, and score patients on the absence or presence of these factors.

A well known and well used pressure sore risk rating scale is the Norton Score, developed for use with elderly patients in 1962. It is a numerical scoring system on five criteria: physical condition, mental state, activity, mobility and incontinence (diagram 3). A score of 14 or less indicates that a patient is at risk of developing sores; people scoring below 12 are considered especially at risk. Other risk calculators frequently used by nurses are: The Waterlow Scale, the Douglas Scale and the Pressure Sore Prediction Score.

Prevention

When patients at risk have been identified, preventive action must be taken. The main aim is relief of pressure, however it is caused. The traditional method of pressure relief is regular changing of the patient's position (at least every two hours). This applies to patients sitting in chairs as well as those in bed. Activities such as turning patients from side to side in bed, lifting them off the bed, helping them to take short walks, even simply standing up, can all help to relieve pressure.

Other factors that help prevent pressure sores are **improved nutrition**, especially increased protein in the diet, increased **mobility**, and pain relief.

Pain relief is particularly important because when patients are in pain they are often tense and reluctant to move. This can increase their risk of developing a pressure sore. All patients need to be assessed for pain and appropriate pain relieving measures introduced when necessary. These pain relieving measures can include complementary therapies such as massage and aromatherapy as well as medicines.

Barrier creams are thought to have a limited role in preventing superficial sores developing, and they should only be used to give protection from friction, dehydration, grazing and damage to the skin from urine or faeces. However, *massaging*

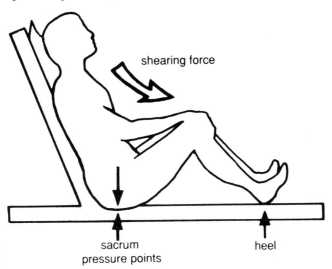

Diagram 2: Pressure points.

the skin with these creams to promote circulation is a misguided practice. Rubbing or vigorously massaging the skin will cause tissues to break down and *increase* the likelihood of a pressure sore developing.

Washing with soap and water as a method of pressure sore prevention is also *an ineffective and potentially harmful practice.* Excessive washing lowers the acidity of the skin and removes the skin's protective substances, making pressure sore formation a greater possibility. Special soaps and cleaners are now available which do not reduce the acidity of the skin and these can be used on incontinent patients who may require frequent washing.

Aids and equipment

When measures such as these are not possible or are impractical, there are a number of aids available that aim to minimise the forces that cause damage. However, it is important to note that any aid which reduces pressure due to compression may not reduce pressure due to shearing forces, and vice versa. For example, sheepskins placed under the sacrum and heels may minimise the damage caused by shearing in sliding down the bed, but will do nothing at all for the pressure caused by compression.

One of the primary causes of compression damage is the type of surface on which the person is placed. A major culprit here is the hospital-type mattress, because in many positions the bodyweight is supported by limited body contact with the flat, firm surface of the hospital bed. Ideally the support surface should have total contact with the body to enable the pressure to be more evenly spread.

Because of the need to spread body weight over a large surface area it is often better to look after someone lying on their back or front, with only limited time, not more than two hours, being spent lying on their sides at any one time. By taking this factor into account people can often be allowed four hours absolutely flat on their backs overnight, thus giving them a better chance to have uninterrupted sleep.

There are a variety of substances that can help body weight to be distributed more evenly. The most well known of these are air and water. Air and water are used to suspend the body on a support surface, and the principle of suspension allows the body weight to be spread over a large surface area.

There are a number of pressure relieving aids that have been designed with this factor in mind: these include special beds and mattresses, cushions and heel pads. Although many of these aids have not been fully evaluated, the principles upon which they are manufactured appear sound and thus they should act to reduce pressure if they are used correctly.

Pressure relieving devices are costly and it is important that they are used properly and effectively. Manufacturers usually provide detailed advice about the use and care of equipment and this should be followed for the best results.

One often-used aid which does not, in fact, have any pressure relieving effect is the ring cushion. These placed under the sacrum are far more likely to cause pressure sores than to relieve them. This is because where the ring is in contact with the body, pressures are increased not decreased. Someone left sitting on a ring cushion for long periods of time will develop a ring of pressure damage where the body is in contact with the ring.

Treatment of sores

If, despite preventive efforts, someone develops a sore, then a positive approach to treatment is required. Pressure sores are now usually classified into five stages. In stages 1 and 2, the skin is red but not broken. The redness of the skin indicates that tissue damage is occurring and will get worse if not treated. In stage 3 the skin is broken and there is usually a small ulcer. In stage 4, the ulcer has become larger and deeper, and in stage 5 the sore is usually infected with areas of dead skin, yellow discharge and an offensive smell.

Treatment of a pressure sore depends upon its stage of development. Pressure sores at stage 1 and stage 2 seldom require more than the prevention measures mentioned earlier. However, pressure sores of grade 3 and above are classed as wounds and a qualified nurse should always supervise treatment. Nevertheless knowledge of the principles involved is useful to all staff.

Knowledge about wound healing is increasing and earlier thoughts about the best way to treat wounds have altered. In the past a dry wound was thought to be best for healing. However, it has now been established that drying a wound delays skin re-growth.

In fact, wound healing occurs two or three times faster when wounds are covered with a dressing which closely covers the wound but allows the oxygen through, compared with wounds covered with conventional dry dressings. These dressings are rather like clingfilm and are designed to retain the fluid produced by the wound and so create a moist wound environment.

Opsite is perhaps the best known of these: this dressing permits the exchange of oxygen and carbon dioxide, and the passage of water vapour, but will not allow bacteria, viruses or water to pass through. These dressings should not be used on infected wounds.

The use of stoma products (primarily designed for people with colostomies) to promote pressure sore healing can be effective. They also retain wound fluid on the wound surface, and so create a moist wound environment.

Another factor important to wound healing is that the wound needs to be at body temperature for healing to take place. Carrying out a dressing and using cold lotions can reduce wound temperature so much that it can take several hours to return to body temperature. For this reason all lotions should be kept at room temperature if possible, and the wound dressing should be disturbed as little as possible.

The choice of dressings available is increasing all the time. When ward staff are not sure what to use, they should seek help from a wound care specialist nurse.

Your role

One way or another, health care assistants are bound to become involved with pressure sores, either by trying to prevent them occurring or helping to treat them if they have occurred. The most important point to remember is that all patients need to change their position regularly, This applies to patients who are sitting in chairs as well as those confined to bed.

On most wards, patients who have any degree of restricted mobility will be assessed for "pressure sore risk" using a recognised assessment tool such as the Norton Score shown on the opposite page. The responsibility for doing this assessment lies with the nursing staff. The score, together with a plan of care for dealing with that problem (or potential problem) will be written in the patient's nursing care plan. Care assistants should be aware of their patients' scores, understand what they mean and then familiarise themselves with the required plans of care for each patient.

When washing and dressing patients, care assistants should always note the condition of vulnerable pressure points such as the sacrum (base of the spine), buttocks and heels. Any signs of redness should be noted and reported.

The treatment of a pressure sore depends on its grading. Because Grades 1 & 2 pressure sores require little more than the standard preventive measures, care assistants will be involved with treating these sores. Pressure sores in which the skin is broken and which may also be infected will be treated by the nursing staff. In between, there are sores which may need some kind of protective covering, for example when the skin is red or slightly grazed. In some situations, care assistants will be shown how to apply these protective dressings.

Points to remember

DO
1. Make sure all patients change their position regularly.
2. Observe patients' skin and report any signs of pressure damage to the patient's nurse.
3. Leave a clean wound alone, covered with a dressing.
4. Encourage a good diet with plenty of protein.
5. Follow each patient's care plan exactly.

DON'T
1. Rub or massage skin vigorously, with or without creams.
2. Wash skin excessively.

NVQ Levels 2 & 3 Core Units
U5 Obtain, transmit and store information relating to the delivery of a care service.

Level 2 Direct Care Endorsement
Z6 Enable clients to maintain and improve their mobility.
z7 Contribute to the movement and treatment of clents.
Z9 Enable clients to maintain their personal hygiene and appearance.
Z19 Enable clients to achieve physical comfort.

Level 3 Acute Care Endorsement
X19 Prepare and undertake agreed ongoing clinical activities with clients in acute care settings.

Physical condition		Mental state		Activity		Mobility		Incontinence	
Good	4	Alert	4	Ambulant	4	Full	4	Not	4
Fair	3	Apathetic	3	Walks with help	3	Slightly limited	3	Occasional	3
Poor	2	Confused	2	Chair-bound	2	Very limited	2	Usually urine	2
Very bad	1	Stuporous	1	Bedfast	1	Immobile	1	Double	1

The Norton Score for pressure sore risk assessment.

CHAPTER 9

Promoting continence

Helen White

• How we all feel about bladder and bowel control • Passing urine • How the bowel works • What is continence and how is it achieved? • Problems that can lead to incontinence • Assessing the type of incontinence • Incontinence of faeces • Toileting programmes • Personal protection • Catheter care and hygiene

Going to the lavatory is a basic human activity which we all perform several times a day without much thought and rarely discuss unless something goes wrong. Our culture seems to find it hard to cope with anything to do with bladders and bowels: the public are embarrassed by the subject, many professionals tend to ignore the problems, and too often care assistants are left to cope with the tasks as best they can.

This chapter will discuss how patients and care staff feel about this sensitive and intimate part of care; explain how continence is achieved and maintained; describe what may go wrong, how incontinence can be managed, and what resources are available.

Confusing terms

Continence is not an easy subject to talk about. It is hard to find words that are descriptive and easy to use, so we often use euphemisms such as "relieving yourself", but these terms can also cause confusion and embarrassment. Nurses and doctors resort to clinical terms which are little understood by most people.

Bladder and bowel control is one of the first skills we learn as a child, and we are taught to use the toilet in private. On admission to hospital it suddenly becomes a public affair. People will go to extraordinary lengths to hide their incontinence, either denying there is a problem and refusing to seek help, or isolating themselves from families and friends. Feelings of shame, helplessness, rejection and misery are commonly expressed.

Our feelings

It is generally assumed that care staff are at ease with all aspects of toileting and incontinence, but we can be just as embarrassed as anyone else at having to assist patients perform these intimate tasks. We too can feel disgusted that someone is not able to control their bladder or bowel, and be resentful that we have to deal with the mess and the smell.

It is important to recognise these feelings and be aware of the effects of social and cultural influences on our lives. Society expects continence to be maintained once it is achieved, isolating or rejecting those who are incontinent.

Ignorance and misunderstanding often

cause unnecessary distress. The word incontinence conjures up images of institutions full of old or disabled people and the stench of urine.

The fact is that incontinence can happen at all ages: children who wet the bed, young women who leak when they sneeze and men who are anxious about their prostate problems.

Patients in hospital are especially at risk. Everyone on the ward has an important part to play in the promotion of continence: as care assistant you are closest to the patient, the person they confide in, the one who performs the most intimate tasks. Talking to patients with knowledge and confidence will give them the reassurance that they are not alone and the guidance to where help is available; but it is equally important that you are also able to share your own feelings and experiences with other staff.

Passing urine

Urine is produced in the kidneys. There are two kidneys situated in the lower part of the back on either side of the spine. They act as a filter and remove waste products from the blood. These, in the form of urine, pass down two tubes, ureters, into the bladder. The bladder is an "elastic" bag made of muscle which expands to store the urine and contracts to squeeze the urine out through a narrow tube, the urethra, which is 4cm long in women, 20cm in men. The bladder and urethra are supported in position by a band of muscles, the pelvic floor muscles.

When the bladder fills to about 250-350mls, it sends messages to the nerves in the lower part of the spine. These messages travel up the spine to the brain. The brain responds by sending the appropriate message back to the bladder. If the time and place are convenient, the

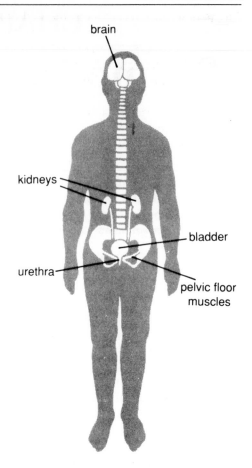

nerves send the messages back down the spine to the bladder muscles. The bladder muscles contract, the urethra relaxes and the urine is squeezed out.

If the time and place are not convenient it is possible to ignore the desire to pass urine, and it will fade from consciousness. Then it returns at intervals until the need is so urgent that emptying can no longer be delayed.

How the bowel works

In normal bowel action, the formed stool is pushed into the lower part of the bowel, called the rectum, by contraction of the muscular walls of the bowel. This triggers sensory receptors in the wall of the rectum which are felt as a desire to empty the bowel. The ring of muscle controlling the anus (the back passage outlet) is relaxed if the time and place is convenient, and the stool is passed, sometimes with the assistance of the muscles of the abdomen.

In a normal bowel action the stool should be soft, well formed and easy to pass. Little hard pellets can indicate constipation.

What is continence?

Continence is being able to pass urine or faeces voluntarily in a socially acceptable place. That is: recognising the need to go; holding on until it is convenient and comfortable; identifying the correct place; then emptying the bladder or bowel completely.

This requires a urinary and bowel system which is working effectively; a nervous system which can convey messages; the ability to move independently or at will, and toilet facilities which are easy to reach and acceptable.

Successful toilet training requires normal physical development, especially of the nervous system, and certain social skills such as being able to remove and replace clothing as necessary at the lavatory; being able to get up and walk to the lavatory, or ask to be taken, or ask for the lavatory; and being able to plan ahead for the lavatory whether the bladder is full or not.

Going to the lavatory demands a complex sequence of events:

• recognising the need to empty the bladder or bowel – so there must be no interruption in the nerve pathway between the bladder and the control centre in the brain

• holding on until an appropriate place is reached, even if the bladder is full (this can be particularly difficult for dependent patients who may have to wait some time for a helper)

• adjusting clothing – undoing zips, pulling down pants

• sitting or standing at the lavatory, initiating the urine stream (or bowel movement) and sustaining it until the bladder or bowel is empty

• wiping the bottom or shaking the penis (it is very important for little girls to be taught to wipe from front to back to avoid the risk of infection)

• flushing the lavatory and making sure it is clean (no urine dribbles on the seat or soiling on the bowl)

• replacing clothes correctly and washing hands before leaving the bathroom.

It is also a very exhausting activity for people who have walking and handling difficulties or tire easily, and patients with heart problems, arthritis or multiple sclerosis.

At what age is continence achieved?

Continence is seen as a major milestone of normal child development. All babies automatically empty their bladder and bowel when they are full, as a reflex action. The age of achieving control varies according to the child's physical and social development and cultural background. The accepted sequence is bowel control by night followed by bowel control by day; bladder control by day followed by bladder control at night. At two years 50 per cent of children will have acquired bowel control and most will have bladder control during the day by three years and night control by four years. At around 18 months there is an awareness of the bladder and a brief holding of urine, and at three years a holding on for longer periods with an increasing bladder capacity. Between the ages of three and four the child should be able to initiate the stream when sitting on the lavatory, and by six years should be able to voluntarily start a stream without a full bladder. Girls generally acquire control before boys. People with learning disabilities can become continent, although they may have to rely on prompting.

What are the problems?

The following questions will highlight the physical, emotional and environmental factors essential to maintaining continence:

Can they recognise the need to go?
Children with spina bifida and adults who are confused may not get the message and there are occasions when both they and others need reminding, for instance little boys holding on to their penis, or older people who are becoming restless. This will be discussed further under toileting programmes.

Can they ask to go?
Young children may use family words such as "poo-poo" to express their need to go to the toilet. Adults who have lost their speech following a stroke may have a special way of communicating; patients who have severe learning difficulties may communicate in a sign language. It is always advisable to check with family or friends to save embarrassment and distress.

Do they know where the lavatory facilities are?
Clear directions which are reinforced with signs will assist patients in their independence. Some patients may prefer or find it easier to use a commode or urine bottle. Whenever possible encourage patients to sit on the lavatory

or commode as this is less stressful and more efficient than a bedpan. With guidance, each individual should make their own choice. Remember to give instructions on how to use urine bottles. Although they are familiar to you, for many people this will be their first experience of hospital and they may be too embarrassed to ask.

Can they get there in time?
The toilet area should be within 10 metres of the day and bed area, and easy to reach. If your patient has walking problems and is slow it may be important that their bed or chair is as close to the door as possible. Shoes and a walking aid may help. If despite all this they often don't get there in time, it is better to wheel them to the lavatory if necessary, and allow them to walk back slowly rather than allow them to suffer the humiliation of wetting on the way.

Care should be taken to ensure that the entrances to the toilet are free from obstruction and not used as an extra storage place, causing added delay.

Can they manage their clothing?
Easy-to-adjust clothing, such as an extended fly with dabs of velcro on trousers and pyjamas, will overcome the difficulty for men of getting the penis out quickly enough, and women may find a fuller skirt where the back can be tucked into the belt, and split-crotch or French knickers quicker if there are problems with handling. Shoes give more support than slippers for easier walking.

Is the lavatory seat at an appropriate height?
The correct position is to sit with the bottom and back well supported and feet firmly on the ground. Little girls can be particularly scared about falling into the bowl, and many people crouch so as not to touch the seat for fear of infection.

In some cultures it is customary to squat with the feet on the seat. Do make sure that the seat and any surrounding rails are secure and able to take this unusual distribution of weight.

Patients who have difficulties balancing, or getting on and off the lavatory, will find aids such as grab rails helpful. The occupational therapist will advise on the positioning of the rails. Patients who need to push themselves up off the loo will require horizontal rails, while those who pull themselves up will need a vertical rail. A foot rest, and if necessary straps to support the trunk, give extra security and confidence. A raised seat is helpful for patients with stiff joints, and men with prostate problems may find sitting a more effective way of emptying their bladder.

Is the lavatory acceptable?

None of us enjoys using a strange lavatory especially in public place and hospital is no exception. Fears of being seen, heard or smelt are common to us all. A clean, well-lit, warm and ventilated lavatory with a door which will shut easily and lock, is a standard all patients should expect. It is important that there is a call system such as a bell so they can be left safely in private.

Trying to pass water and even worse having a bowel movement, when you are aware someone can hear and smell you, is most inhibiting. These problems can be overcome by running water, lining the pan with paper and spraying with a deodoriser.

Are the cleaning facilities adequate?

Most people are worried about the risk of infection when using hospital lavatories. Providing dispensers containing disposable lavatory covers, which can be flushed away, can be a great help. Holders containing soft lavatory paper

should be positioned on either side of the lavatory to accommodate people who have limited use of their hands. Special easy-to-hold bottom wipers, which have extended tongs to hold a large tissue, or a combined lavatory/bidet which automatically sprays warm water followed by warm air, may be available. These do give independence, but careful instructions and reassurance are needed. They can be quite frightening to young children and older people.

Patients who are soiled through faecal incontinence should be cleaned as soon as possible. Gently remove the faecal matter using a large soft tissue or special wipe, then wash with warm water and dry thoroughly. If the soiling has dried on to the skin, cleansing agents which can be sprayed on to the skin and then wiped off with a moist tissue are very helpful, particularly where the skin is already fragile.

Urine is acid and can cause skin soreness, which in turn can lead to rashes and infection. Avoid scented soap and talcum powder as these can add to the irritation. A flannel for washing face and hands should be kept separately from the one used for washing between the legs. If the skin is particularly sensitive, patting between the legs with a soft towel or drying with a cool hairdryer can be helpful. Nursing staff will advise you on skin and barrier creams.

People from certain cultures, such as Moslems and Sikhs, hold strong views about personal hygiene, and may for example require a special jug so they can wash with running water. If in doubt it is best to ask family or friends.

How much are they drinking?

Many older people believe they should drink less so that less urine will be passed. What happens, though, is that the urine becomes concentrated, the bladder capacity may become smaller and other problems can result, including constipation. A good guide is six cups of fluid for children and 10 cups for adults over 24 hours. Do encourage more water and less tea, coffee and cola, as these drinks stimulate the kidneys.

Parents often teach their children to go to the lavatory each time they go to the shops, school or a journey. This habit of going at every opportunity trains the bladder to empty at a low volume and often persists throughout adulthood so these people will never venture far from a public toilet. Anyone who requires to pass urine more than every two hours or who gets up more than twice a night, unless they are on medication, requires investigation.

Bowel frequency is very individual – once a day, twice a week – what is important is the *consistency*, not frequency. Stools should be soft, formed and easy to pass; straining to pass a stool can indicate constipation.

Certain medicines, such as water tablets (diuretics) increase the amount of urine, sometimes very rapidly, so there is little warning. Sleeping tablets (sedatives) can delay the message being relayed and responded to by the brain; pain killers (analgesics) can cause constipation.

What is their attitude to continence?
We are all anxious when we are in an unfamiliar situation and hospital can be one of the most stressful. Children and adults may wet themselves on admission, which may be acceptable for the child, but not so for the older person. This humiliating experience is a memory which will never fade.

Depression can affect children as well as older people, and may lead to a loss of motivation. This should not be confused with laziness and attention-seeking. Loss of independence can lead some patients to use bladder and bowel control to their advantage; for many it is the only means they have left to express themselves. Forcing patients to the lavatory can have the opposite effect to the one you want.

Incontinence

Incontinence means the uncontrolled (involuntary) loss of urine or faeces. It is not a disease but is a symptom of an underlying problem which can happen to anyone at any time of life. It affects more women than men but it is not an inevitable consequence of old age or disability. Indeed the majority of old people remain continent all their lives.

Incontinence at any age causes physical, emotional, social and financial hardship and severely disrupts people's lives. Many see incontinence in older people as a natural stage of regression to infancy and treat them accordingly, increasing dependence and loss of adult status.

There are many causes of incontinence and an individual can suffer from several symptoms. Treatment or management must be based on individual assessment and investigation to discover the type of incontinence and possible causes.

Assessment

Assessment is based on answers to questions such as the following:

Do you leak when you cough or sneeze?
Leaking of urine on exertion, **stress incontinence**, can occur when there is extra strain on the tummy, such as coughing or sneezing. It is a common complaint in women of all ages, who have weakened muscles around the bladder and urethra during pregnancy and childbirth, after the menopause and if there is a history of constipation.

It can be cured by exercises, correctly done, to strengthen these muscles, and in extreme cases by surgery to tighten the muscles. It can be successfully managed by not letting the bladder become over-full, avoiding constipation, doing pelvic floor exercises, and wearing protective garments.

Do you have to go frequently and quickly?
A strong need to pass urine quickly and often, sometimes not reaching the lavatory in time because the bladder muscles become overactive and contract with little warning, is known as **urge incontinence.** The person rushes to the lavatory immediately they are aware of their bladder in an effort to prevent urine loss. The bladder seldom holds more than a few millilitres of urine because it is emptied so frequently. This quickly becomes a habit, and the time between emptyings becomes less and less – in extreme cases every 15 minutes.

It is common to men and women, particularly those who have problems affecting the nervous system, such as multiple sclerosis or stroke, those with dementia, and children and adults who are bedwetters. Sometimes people become so depressed and anxious about having an accident that they refuse to be far from a lavatory.

This type of incontinence is particularly common in older people who are admitted to hospital. Again it is curable in many cases, by introducing a programme of bladder exercises to extend the intervals between trips to the lavatory, and wearing light protective garments to gain confidence. Medicines to quieten the bladder muscles may also be prescribed.

Do you have to get up at night?
Dribbling or continuous leakage of urine, sometimes leading to wetting the bed at night, is known as **overflow incontinence**. It is often associated with an obstruction at the bladder neck, such as an enlarged prostate gland (in men) or constipation. It may be due to the bladder muscles not contracting properly, for example where there is damage to the nerves of the spinal chord, so the bladder does not empty completely, retaining a substantial volume of urine which causes a feeling of fullness even after urine has been passed.

If left untreated this can lead to repeated urinary infections and other serious complications, so a medical assessment is important. How the condition is managed will depend on the cause, but always check for constipation and provide personal and bed protection to preserve the patient's comfort and dignity. In some cases an intermittent or indwelling catheter (see page 74) will be recommended.

Do you find you get no warning?
The bladder may empty without any warning – **reflex incontinence** – because the nervous system is not conveying the messages to the brain. This may happen following spinal injury, extreme confusion or fear, or in children following an accident or acute illness.

In some cases a chart recording the times of the reflex can indicate a pattern which will allow toileting at set intervals to anticipate the loss, or it may be necessary for the urine to be contained with highly absorbent pads or another recommended method.

Can you get there in time?
Simply not getting to the lavatory in time because of walking and handling difficulties – **functional incontinence** – can usually be managed with easy-to-wear clothing, commodes and urine bottles as appropriate.

Incontinence of faeces

Loss of either solid or runny unformed stools, or soiling of clothing, is referred to as faecal incontinence. Although this is not nearly as common as urinary incontinence it can be far more distressing because of the resulting mess and smell. The most common cause is severe constipation, which can happen in children as well as adults, when a hard mass of stool forms in the the lower part of the bowel. Liquid stool trickles past the blockage as a continual faecal loss, causing soiling of clothes and bedding. This is called **constipation with overflow**. It has a very distinctive smell and should not be confused with soiling because the child or adult has not been able to clean themselves, or diarrhoea due to tummy upset or allergy.

There are many causes: embarrassment at using a strange lavatory, poor diet including insufficient fluids, lack of exercise, certain medicines, difficulty in passing hard lumps or a solid mass, orand an interruption of the nerve messages to the brain such as occurs in spinal injury or spina bifida.

The simple management is to avoid the situation by ensuring that the toilets are acceptable, the diet is adequate, and a routine is established. The best time for a bowel movement is very individual but after a meal or hot drink, when the gut has been stimulated, is often good.

Bulking and softening agents, suppositories, and in extreme cases an enema to clear out the bowel, may be necessary. It will be a medical or nursing decision, but you have an important part in contributing to this.

Young children can find constipation very frightening and upsetting as well as painful if the stool is particularly hard or large. They may try to prevent themselves having a bowel movement or may well use this as a means of attracting attention. Whatever the reason it is important that the situation is treated in the early stages.

In the ageing bowel the sphincter muscles may become lax and less efficient, or there may be a lifetime of straining to open the bowels or a persistent use of laxatives which contribute to the loss of control. In most cases the symptoms can be treated. New techniques in surgery can sometimes improve the function of the muscles controlling the back passage, which may have been damaged at birth or as the result of an injury.

If protective garments are necessary they should be snug fitting to avoid seepage. Special attention must be given to skin care and personal hygiene; in severe cases it may be necessary to provide a deodorising agent to maintain the patient's dignity.

Bowels are a very private affair and should be dealt with discreetly. Fortunately the old routine of asking patients in a loud voice if they have had their bowels opened, has gone from hospital wards.

Toileting programme

Toileting is the term applied to the intervals when patients should visit or be taken to the lavatory to maintain bladder and bowel control. The programme will depend on several factors including the bladder function, mental ability and mobility of the patient. Patients must be assessed as individuals so that the most appropriate programme can be introduced.

Toileting cannot be imposed on an unwilling or uncooperative patient, even if they are intellectually competent. It is therefore important that patient and staff alike are convinced that success is achievable.

The assessment will include keeping accurate charts of the times urine is passed in each 24 hours, and the amount if possible. This record should be kept for five to seven days so that a pattern may emerge on which to base the programme. This requires the motivation and cooperation of all staff as well as the patient. Whenever possible encourage the patient to fill in the record themselves. Many commercial companies provide simple easy-to-record charts and children have great fun creating their own imaginative charts.

It is important that both patients and staff understand what is expected of them, and then stick to the programme.

Set interval toileting is reminding or taking the patient to the toilet. It does not teach independence but is useful for people who forget, have no bladder sensation or have no regular pattern of passing urine.

Individualised toileting is working out when the patient is most likely to pass urine, by following the chart you made, and then reminding, or taking them to the lavatory 15 minutes before wetting may occur, and adjusting the time interval as necessary.

Bladder retraining is a programme to extend the intervals between going to pass urine. The aim is to hold on for two- to three-hourly intervals. It is useful for people who have lost their confidence and go just in case, but it does need much understanding and support for patient and helper.

Personal protection

Sometimes it may be necessary to provide protective garments or appliances for patients who are not able to be completely dry or who are awaiting treatment.

There are thousands of aids available which can make selection difficult. The final choice of product must be made by the patient whenever possible, but the type of product will depend on the nature of the incontinence – urinary, faecal or both; the quantity of loss – leak, gush or soiling; the personal details of the patient including sex, dexterity, mobility and mental ability.

If reusables are to be tried the laundry facilities need to be flexible to allow for the manufacturer's washing instructions. The availability of the product once the patient goes home is most important.

You should aim to become as familiar as possible with the products used, their application and management, so that you can advise and support your patient and relatives as well as provide a high quality of care. Too often aids are inappropriate, or are used incorrectly because of ignorance or lack of instruction. This can be costly to the patient's dignity as well as your time and the resources of the unit.

The continence adviser can advise on selection, although this is often restricted by cost and hospital purchasing policies. Some products are expensive for regular use if bought independently.

Pads and pants

Absorbent garments and pads are the most commonly used, and reusable products are becoming popular for people who have a long term urinary loss. They are not recommended for a faecal loss because of staining and washing difficulties. An absorbent aid is designed to keep a patient comfortable and free from leakage for 3-4 hours.

For men and women who have a light loss, machine washable pants with an absorbent gusset can give a feeling of confidence. Where the loss is more severe, there is a range of disposable or reusable liners which can be worn inside the person's own pants.

Body worn liners should be cupped to form a gully, with the absorbent surface facing upwards and kept in position with close fitting pants. Pants and all-in-one garments should be selected by hip fitting. Check the manufacturer's instructions if you are unsure.

Sheaths: Men may prefer to wear an appliance such as a disposable sheath, which should remain in position for 24 hours. There are other appliances which can be worn for longer periods. Little boys and older men who have a retracted penis may have difficulty in keeping these on and should be offered an alternative.

Sheets: There are also highly absorbent washable bed sheets which can help to improve sleep patterns because they keep the person warm and dry. It is important to follow the manufacturer's instructions to obtain the maximum benefit.

Catheter care

Sometimes a hollow tube called a catheter is placed in the bladder in order to drain the urine away. A catheter may be used once and then removed (intermittent catheterisation) or left in position to drain continuously and changed at intervals (indwelling catheter).

Intermittent catheterisation is passing a fine, usually plastic, catheter through the urethra into the bladder to completely drain it of urine at regular intervals. Children can be taught at a very early age and likewise for adults old age is no barrier, but sight, dexterity and willingness are important.

This method of bladder control has revolutionised the lives of people of all ages who had previously suffered repeated urinary infections and had their lifestyle severely restricted. It is suitable for patients whose bladder is unable to empty completely for some reason, such as children with spina bifida and adults with multiple sclerosis. Whenever possible the patient is encouraged to catheterise themselves, so that they are more independent.

The indwelling catheter is passed in to the bladder, usually through the urethra, but sometimes directly into the bladder via the abdomen. It is made of a latex or silicone material, depending on the length of time it is to remain in the bladder, and is attached to a drainage bag, which collects the urine. It is important always to ensure that the connecting tubing is not kinked or compressed so that the urine can flow freely, and that the bag is below the level of the bladder, as urine cannot flow uphill.

The bag can be supported by leg straps or a garment such as a pouch sewn on to the leg of underpants or trousers. The method of support is important as it not only assists in the drainage but also in the dignity of the patient. No one likes to see bags of urine and many patients do not want their family and friends to know this intimate aspect of their care.

Patients and relatives can find the prospect of a catheter daunting and you may find yourself having to allay their fears, by explaining clearly so they understand the reasons and the care of the system. Most of the catheter manufacturers provide excellent patient guides.

Any indication of infection, such as the patient feeling ill or having a raised temperature, should be reported to nursing staff immediately.

Hygiene guidelines

• Always wash hands before as well as after emptying the drainage bag.

- Never proceed from patient to patient emptying their drainage bags (because of the risk of cross infection).
- Attach the night bag to the leg bag rather than changing one to the other.
- Never allow the tap of the drainage bag to touch the floor.
- Pay special attention to personal hygiene, washing between the legs at least twice a day.
- Ensure that the catheter and drainage tube are draining freely, and there is no blockage.
- The bag should slope towards the tap to allow complete emptying.
- Support and maintain the shape of the bag using a garment or straps. Remember legs can become swollen by evening so check straps have not become too tight, or hang the bag on a stand on the wheelchair or bed.

Points to remember

1. You are central in reassuring patients that their problems are recognised and will be given sympathetic help.
2. Your knowledge will give you the confidence to encourage patients to talk about their problems. Ask senior staff if you feel unsure about a query or problem.
3. Bladder and bowel control (continence) is a skill we learn in early life and normally retain till the end.
4. Losing this control – incontinence – is a very common problem, especially for patients in hospital.
5. The symptoms are embarrassing for patients and care workers alike. It is not an easy subject to talk about: recognising your own feelings is important.
6. Incontinence is a symptom which has many causes.
7. Incontinence can often be cured, and always improved.
8. Success depends on the accurate recording and reporting of your observations to the team.
9. Treatment is a team effort involving the patient, their family and all ward staff

Resources

A Guide to Continence Assessment and Bladder Retraining. Produced by Di Lofting, St Martin's Hospital, Bath. An easy to read practical guide.

Equipment for Disabled People: *Personal care – adults* and *Children with disabilities.* Illustrated details of selected equipment. Mary Marlborough Lodge, Nuffield Orthopaedic Centre, Headington, Oxford OX3 7LD. Tel: 0865 750103.

Incontinence Advisory Service, The Disabled Living Foundation, 380-384 Harrow Rd, London W9 2HU. Tel: 071 289 6111.

NVQ Levels 2 & 3 Value Base Units

Oa Promote anti-discriminatory practice.
Oc Promote and support individual rights and choice within service delivery.
Od Acknowledge individuals' personal beliefs and identity
Oe Support individuals through effective communication.

Levels 2 & 3 Core Unit

U5 Obtain, transmit and store information relating to the delivery of a care service.

Level 2 Direct Care Endorsement

Z6 Enable clients to maintain and improve their mobility.
Z9 Enable clients to maintain their personal hygiene and appearance.
Z11 Enable clients to access and use toilet facilities.

Level 3 Acute Care Endorsement

Z12 Contribute to the management of client continence.
X19 Prepare and undertake agreed ongoing clinical activities with clients in acute care settings.

CHAPTER 10

Black people and equal opportunities

Peter Ferns

• What is racism? What is race equality? • Some good and bad ways we can respond to racism • Challenging stereotypes • Valuing cultural diversity • Maintaining self-esteem and confidence • Equal opportunities

Because of racism in our society, Black people are an oppressed group who experience discrimination and disadvantage in their everyday lives. So in caring for them their experiences must be taken into account, and services must both challenge racism and work to stop racism happening.

"Black" is used as a political term to stand for solidarity or togetherness for people who experience racism because of their skin colour. By using the term "Black", it is hoped to give people support and confidence to stand up against racism and not feel isolated. It is spelled here with a capital letter to remind us that it is a political term and not just a reference to colour.

What is racism ?

Racism is a word to describe racial *prejudice*, that is negative attitudes and beliefs about Black people, and racial *discrimination*, which is unfair behaviour towards a group of people because of their skin colour. Thus it involves the abuse of power by white people, who have more power in a society which has

been racist for a long time, and has taken power away from Black people in many different ways.

Racism can be experienced on two levels: between individuals, or from institutions and organisations in society such as education, housing authorities, the legal system, health and social services. There is a great deal of evidence that racism is still a big problem for Black people in Britain today.

What is race equality ?

Race equality involves changing white people's negative attitudes towards Black people, introducing ways of thinking about people which value their racial and cultural differences. A second aspect of race equality is to put into place equal opportunities policies and other measures to deal with institutional discrimination and safeguard Black people's rights to fair treatment by those organisations. The third aspect of race equality is to empower Black people, which means to support Black people in taking more control over their own lives and working against racism in society.

Responding to racism

How do white people, and organisations run mainly by white people, respond to racism? The following are examples of unhelpful responses often made when racism and racist practices are challenged:

• **"It's not my concern."** This comes from a belief that racism is the concern of Black people, and is not really to do with white people's attitudes and behaviour. So, for instance, people mistakenly believe that racism can only happen if you have Black people present.

• **"Black people should fit into British culture."** This assumes that British culture is only white and European, not the mix of cultures it actually is. It is also another way of saying that white British culture is best and that white people have nothing to learn from other cultures.

• **"There's no racism here."** This comes from a reluctance to accept the unpleasant reality that Britain still has a racist society which treats Black people unfairly. Racism is bound to affect every organisation in this country because it is part of so many things in society.

• **"I treat everyone the same."** This is a colour-blind approach which does not accept the real life experiences of Black people who *are* treated differently. "The same" often means being treated as if you are white. Anyway, equality does not mean being treated the same, it means equal respect for people's rights, experiences and their individual needs.

• **"I need to know about Black people's cultures."** There is nothing wrong with wanting to know more about a person's culture but care must be taken not to stereotype and make assumptions about people based on their culture. It is very difficult to fully understand a person's culture. So the best thing to do is to treat the person and their family as experts and to respect the person's culture as an important aspect of their care.

Experiences of racism

Black people experience racism in the following ways:

• Being racially stereotyped because of your skin colour. A stereotype is where a person is assumed to have particular characteristics or behaviours because they belong to an identified group in society. So stereotypes are a barrier to seeing a person as an individual, and to appreciating their individual skills and talents.

• Not having your skills and abilities recognised partly because people around you do not understand your cultural skills and abilities.

• Being seen as negatively different because of your culture.

• Losing self confidence, self esteem, racial and cultural identity and being treated as if you were white.

• Being regarded as less intelligent then you are because you cannot speak English very well.

• Not being listened to; having your wishes and preferences ignored.

• Having people who do not understand your culture decide what is best for you.

• Having your family and community ties weakened when these ties are essential for you to survive racism.

• Being unsure about your rights and how to stand up for them and make a complaint.

• Having to deal with organisations that do not uphold equal rights for Black people.

• Having your views about service quality ignored.

• Not having access to culturally appropriate services.

Working for race equality

Hospitals are there to help people, to treat illness, to enable people to regain self-confidence and gain more control over their lives, and provide personal care in a way that is acceptable to them.

The services offered must meet Black people's needs in a way that does not offend people and suits them in terms of traditions, customs or religious beliefs. If these kinds of changes in services do not happen, health services will continue to be effectively denied to many Black communities and remain inaccessible and inappropriate. In this way services will strengthen racism in society rather than making a valuable contribution to greater race equality.

Nurses and care assistants must also take personal responsibility for their practice if services are to work for race equality. One committed care worker in a workplace can make a great deal of difference to the day-to-day experience of the individuals they work with.

Challenging stereotypes

Clear evidence of stereotyping can be found in written records. For instance, Asian parents may be described as too rigid and interfering in the lives of their adult daughter or son. The way information is recorded and gathered often has a big effect on the assessment of needs and the subsequent services provided. The needs of Black people and their families are often perceived through the eyes of white assessors who have little or no understanding of the family's culture, and have biased attitudes about Black people gained from a racist society.

Evidence of stereotyping can also be found in the way that services treat Black people but this evidence is more difficult to collect. For instance, African Caribbean young men are often perceived as being more "aggressive" and "threaten-ing" by staff, a common stereotype projected by newspapers and TV programmes. In mental health services this has led to Black young men being labelled more readily as having "challenging" behaviours and being placed in more restrictive living situations.

Valuing cultural diversity

The cultures of Black people are portrayed through negative images in many ways, and this makes it even more important for services to carry positive images of Britain as a multicultural society. Black people will feel more comfortable in surroundings that reflect their own cultures in some way such as posters, pictures, books and newspapers. It is also important to respect people's culture in an active way. For instance, by being aware of and helping people to celebrate different festivals, or learning a little about people's different languages and customs.

Maintaining self-confidence

All patients are likely to experience more stress because of temporary or longer-term ill-health. Self-confidence and self-esteem may well be affected adversely. Black patients are even more vulnerable to such stress due to the additional pressures of institutional racism, language and cultural barriers.

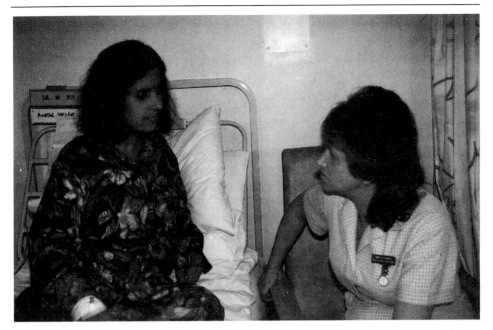

Hospitals must meet people's needs in a way that suits them, their traditions, customs and beliefs.

Hair and skin care

An essential part of personal identity is personal appearance, and for Black people it is important to pay attention to the cultural factors that come into dress, hair and skin care and personal hygiene.

For instance, it is very important for African Caribbean people to have regular combing of their hair with the use of the appropriate hair gels and fashionable hair styles. Failure to do this will result in matted hair in a short period of time, which can quickly necessitate cutting a person's hair in order to comb it properly. Sikhs do not usually have their hair cut but require hair styling to a "top-knot" and the application of special oils.

Skin care for African Caribbean people has also been conspicuously neglected in long-term hospital settings, resulting in dry, flaking skin due to the lack of appropriate skin oils. Information about hair and skin care is available through various publications (see Resource list). Hospitals could make links with local hairdressers and beauticians who specialise in Black hair and skin care.

Food is another aspect of basic care where cultural and religious needs are ignored or inadequately catered for. It is a basic right to have food that is your own choice, but sadly in many hospitals such choice is denied to both Black and white people. The impact on Black people can be worse, because the food offered is neither acceptable to their religion nor culturally familiar. Offering everyone foods from different cultures can be a good way of valuing cultural diversity.

Longer-term institutional care

Where Black people have been in institutional care for a long period of time and have had little or no contact with Black communities or their families, it is likely that they may not have a strong racial or cultural identity and may even have negative feelings towards other Black people. In this situation it is vitally important for staff to help them gain a positive view of their own racial identity and cultural heritage.

Black people should be offered opportunities to learn more about their family's culture, traditions and history of their community. If a Black person does not have English as their first language, it would be necessary for care workers to enable them to communicate in their first language with another person from their community.

Making decisions

People who are not used to being asked about their opinions soon lose the skills to communicate their choices, and may even be afraid of choosing. Hospital staff have to support people in identifying their preferences and making choices.

Knowing your options and making choices also requires power and influence in decisions to bring choices into effect. Hospitals have to be made more sensitive to the views of all patients, giving them more say in the way services assist them and especially in the major decisions that affect their lives.

Equal opportunities

It seems obvious to tell you to read your organisation's Equal Opportunities Policy, but it is surprising the number of people who are not even sure what such policies say. Read the policy then ask questions of your manager if you are unsure about anything.

If you are working for a good organisation, there may also be a Race Equality Strategy, which is a set of plans to put the policy into operation, and practice guidelines which give workers practical ways of using the policy in the workplace. It is the responsibility of every employee of the organisation to put the policy into practice, and workers will have

to think about the type of training they need to bring race equality into their practice. If care staff are unsure about working with Black people, some of the more progressive organisations may have Race Advisers to support and advise staff in practical, "on-the-job" strategies.

Points to remember

1. Racism is still a big problem for Black people in Britain today.
2. Working for race equality involves shanging attitudes, valuing cultural differences and empowering Black people to take more control over their own lives.
3. Look out for discrimination and stereotyping, and challenge it.
4. Try to help Black people in your care maintain their self-esteem with appropriate hair and skin care.

Resources

Afro skin, hair care and recipes - booklet from the Commission for Racial Equality, and *Hair Care* by Carol Baxter, National Extension College for Training in Health and Race. Also available from CRE.

Black Beauty and Hair magazine, available from bookshops or Hawker Publications, 13 Park House, 140 Battersea Park Road, London SW11 4NB.

NVQ Levels 2 & 3 Value Base Units

Oa Promote anti-discriminatory practice.
Oc Promote and support individual rights and choice within service delivery.
Od Acknowledge individuals' personal beliefs and identity.
Oe Support individuals through effective communication.

Level 2 Direct Care Endorsement

Z9 Enable clients to maintain their personal hygiene and appearance.
Z10 Enable clients to eat and drink

CHAPTER 11

Caring for people from different cultures

Lynne Swiatczak

• How to help when there are problems in understanding and communication
• Worship and prayer • Diet • Involving relatives • Attitudes to illness and pain
• Physical care • Death and dying • Respect for individuals

When patients are in hospital the emphasis is always on treating each patient as an individual person with their own likes and dislikes, habits and preferences. This is just as important, if not more so, when caring for people from a different cultural background from our own.

It is vital that assessment of each person's needs is carried out on admission and throughout the patient's stay in hospital. Some hospitals employ Ethnic Link Workers, who can be called upon for help and advice at any time.

When patients are from a different culture there are often areas where planning and delivering specific aspects of care is very important. Some of those areas are listed below:

Communication

Some patients may not speak English and therefore have problems in both understanding and communicating. It is important also to realise that not all patients can read their own language.

Gestures and facial expressions can mean different things in different cultures, and so this too should be taken into consideration.

Communication needs affect every aspect of care. Giving information, which we know can lead to greater patient choice, is more difficult. Some hospitals provide standard information in different languages, but if the patient cannot read this is of no benefit.

There are several ways of solving this problem, one of which is using an interpreter. Often a friend or relative is asked to translate for the patient. This can be helpful, but the problem is that there is no way care staff can assess that the information has not been altered in the translation, or that the patient understands the information which has been given. This is vitally important when asking for consent to surgery or other forms of treatment.

There are usually interpreters who work for the hospital, and often doctors and nurses who speak different languages volunteer to translate for patients. Some hospitals have also translated information onto tape in various languages.

While this can all help a great deal, it must be remembered, to quote one example, that all Indian patients do not speak the same language, and that even if they do speak Gujarati or Punjabi, their own dialect may be completely different. The most important thing to remember is to provide some way of checking understanding.

Worship and prayer

Worship and prayer play a vital part in the life of religious people of all faiths. Each patient will have their own specific prayer and worship needs. These can range from requiring a place in which to pray to the provision of religious books and equipment, such as a prayer mat. If these articles are provided there are specific rules and regulations regarding their use and these must be strictly followed.

Finding space for patients to worship can prove difficult in a busy ward but every effort must be made, even if it means using the ward office or treatment room. All staff must be aware of a patient's religious requirements, and must accept that this aspect of their life is very important to their wellbeing.

Some Muslim patients pray regularly several times a day, which can be difficult following surgery or when the patient is on bed rest. On these occasions the patient must be helped to worship in whatever way they can until they are able to continue their usual practices. Their religious leader may be able to give guidance.

Diet

Some religions have specific dietary requirements. For example Hindu followers do not usually eat beef as the cow is considered a sacred animal. It must be remembered, however that not all Hindu patients follow their religion

strictly. Many other cultures have other requirements which may mean they need food served in specific ways. Food for Jewish patients is known as Kosher; it arrives on the ward in sealed containers which must be presented to the patient still sealed, not opened, and transferred onto a plate. The patient will usually use their own cutlery which may be provided in the sealed package.

Muslim patients usually eat Halal meats and these are provided by the catering department of the hospital.

Some patients prefer to have relatives bring food into hospital for them and this should be allowed wherever possible. If this is the case all care staff must ensure that relatives are aware of any specific medical requirements, for example if the patient is diabetic. Food storage and hygiene regulations must also be followed, however, so it is important to discuss this with the patient and their relatives.

Involvement of relatives

In some cultures the patient sees themself as part of a community, which makes some decisions on the patient's behalf. Relatives often have an important role to play in giving care to patients, and must not be forgotten when planning care. Some patients prefer relatives to assist them with their personal hygiene requirements, rather than care staff, and relatives should be allowed, encouraged and helped to do this wherever possible.

Facilities should be provided for relatives to stay at the hospital; this is sometimes preferred, particularly if the patient has communication needs.

Relatives often have specific involvement in decision making. For example an Asian lady may not agree to treatment without her husband's approval.

Planning their own care

Some patients believe that it is the role of the doctor and nurse to plan care and may be quite offended if asked to contribute to their own care planning. All care staff must be aware of the patient's choice in this matter.

Some patients have specific beliefs which may affect their care; staff should be aware of this possibility and seek the relevant information.

Complementary therapies

Many cultures advocate the use of complementary therapies and homeopathic treatments.

When in hospital they should be encouraged to discuss the use of these with medical and nursing staff as many of them are not prohibited but can complement the treatment given (although there are some that should not be used). Many of the treatments previously viewed as alternative, such as acupuncture and aromatherapy, are now used in everyday practice in many hospital.

Illness and pain

Although it is dangerous to generalise, there are cultural influences on people's response to pain and illness. This can be very important when assessing a patient's response to treatment.

We may, for example, assume that analgesics (painkillers) are working when in fact the patient is uncomplaining because they feel they should have to suffer. Other patients react in different ways: some patients may have low pain thresholds and what may seem to us to be minor discomfort may be very acute pain to them.

Physical care

There are many instances where the physical care of the patient is different because of cultural needs.

Many Asian patients do not like to bathe because they see this as sitting in dirty water; they prefer to rinse themselves with clean water. Afro Caribbean people have specific skin and hair care requirements, requiring hair gels and oils in order to prevent their hair becoming matted and their skin dry and sore. There are also many patients who will not allow people of the opposite sex to see them undressed. Many Asian women always cover their hair and their legs. Sikh men always wear turbans and these are not removed.

Death and dying

Each culture has specific requirements. Some religions forbid the washing of a body after death, some require this to be done by relatives, some require specific rituals to be performed by religious leaders at or immediately after the time of death. Each member of staff must be aware of these requirements, as a wrong action can lead to serious consequences for the family and community of the dead person.

Each hospital will have a list of religious leaders and if the patient or family has not requested a specific person, this list should be used to summon the appropriate person at the time of death.

Future care

Decisions relating to future care are often the responsibility of the whole family and/or the wider community. The belief that the family take care of their own is largely a myth in Britain today where many families are separated in different parts of the country. There are still few nursing and residential homes which offer specific care for people of different cultures, whether elderly people or those who are physically or mentally disabled.

Different races

When assessing patients it is important that we remember that it is not only patients with black or brown skin who have different needs. There are growing populations of Chinese, Polish, Ukranian, Turkish, Greek and many other nationalities who all have specific needs. The older population may be more traditional in their beliefs and outlook, but this is not always the case.

Respect for individuals

As always, remember that every patient is an individual: delivering stereotyped care because they are from a certain culture would be as bad as ignoring their cultural needs altogether. Your role in providing care is the same as for any other patient, with a special regard for any specific needs. You must not judge patients because of their beliefs or customs and must always respect those beliefs and traditions.

One of the most important things to remember is that each patient will follow their religion to different degrees. We would not assume that one Baptist would be representative of all Baptists and we should therefore not assume that one Muslim is representative of all Muslims. Each patient will still have their own personal needs, and will have their own way of living their faith.

Communication skills
The communication skills of all care staff should be developed in ongoing training (see Chapter 3, Talking and Listening).

Points to remember

1. Many patients will need help in both understanding and communicating. It is vital to find some way of checking that they have understood important information.
2. Staff must accept and encourage regular worship and prayer where it is important to the individual.
3. Find out about specific requirements for diet and other aspects of care.
4. Everyone is an individual - don't give stereotyped care just because they belong to a certain culture or religion.

Resources
Caring in a Multi-racial Society, by Alix Henley. Bloomsbury and Islington Health Authority, London WC1.
Health Needs of a Multi-racial Population. Liverpool Health Authority Community and Priority Services, Sefton General Hospital, Smithdown Road, Liverpool L15 2HE..

NVQ Levels 2 & 3 Value Base Units
Oa Promote anti-discriminatory practice.
Oc Promote and support individual rights and choice within service delivery.
Od Acknowledge individuals' personal beliefs and identity.
Oe Support individuals through effective communication.

Level 2 Direct Care Endorsement
Z9 Enable clients to maintain their personal hygiene and appearance.
Z10 Enable clients to eat and drink

Level 2 Core Unit
W2 Contribute to the ongoing support of clients and others significant to them.

Level 3 Acute Care Endorsement
Z14 Support clients and others at times of loss.

CHAPTER 12

Care of the dying patient

Sheila Mackie Bailey

• Our experience of death and dying • HIV and AIDS • Cultural differences • Choosing for ourselves • The dying process: denial, anger, bargaining, depression, acceptance • Physical care • Tactics staff use to avoid distress • Staff training and support • Spiritual care • The patient's closest relationship

When caring for a dying person whatever their age – baby, child, adolescent or elderly – your main task is to ensure that they experience an "appropriate" death. By this I mean the kind of death they would have chosen for themselves if they had the opportunity and were able to choose.

The way in which such a preference can be expressed will be discussed later. However, when a person is dying others are affected, especially close relatives, partners, close friends and those who are caring for them.

Experience of dying

Up until very recent times not only did both birth and death take place in the home, but after someone had died the body remained in the house until the funeral. As a result people grew up with first-hand experience of dying and death.

Not only that but the death rate among all age groups was high, either due to infectious disease or conditions for which there was no known cure.

Nowadays things have changed.

Developments in surgical techniques, advances in drug treatments and technological advances have meant that people who might have died even 10 years ago now survive. Improvements in standards of living, healthier diet, lifestyle and living environment, mean that people are living longer than in past generations. In this context death may not be accepted as inevitable in the way that it was, and care staff may well feel a sense of failure when someone dies.

But perhaps a more significant change is the fact that most people die in hospitals or nursing homes. Even if someone dies at home, their body is taken to the undertakers where it remains until the funeral. As a result most of us grow up with little or no experience of dying and death, making it difficult when we first encounter death at work.

HIV and AIDS

Despite medical advances and healthier lifestyle, we do not live in a world free of disease. While diseases such as smallpox have been eradicated, others have

85

evolved. For example HIV (Human Immunodeficiency Virus) and AIDS (Acquired Immune Deficiency Syndrome) are on the increase in the UK and elsewhere. They affect men and women in all walks of life and from many different backgrounds, and may be encountered in any ward of an acute hospital.

HIV and AIDS are related conditions: HIV is the virus which may be present in an infected person's bloodstream long before the disease AIDS develops. One myth which must be dispelled is that HIV and AIDS only affect homosexuals and drug addicts; they also affect heterosexual men and women, babies and children.

People with HIV or AIDS may need treatment for other medical conditions, and thus may to be admitted to any ward of a hospital – surgery, medicine, orthopaedics, gynaecology, paediatrics or maternity. Every hospital has a policy regarding the care of these patients, including precautions which may need to be taken for the protection of staff and the patient, and a statement about staff members' obligation to care for them to the best of their ability.

Many of those dying of AIDS related illnesses have special needs. For their own protection from infection, they must be nursed on an isolation ward, and this may be stressful both for the patient, their partner and their family. Care staff must be very sensitive to this distress, and try to make any necessary precautions as discreet as possible. Where special clothing and masks have to be worn, do not make a fuss about it or complain when the patient or visitors can hear you.

Patients with AIDS related illnesses are likely also to be very sensitive to the reactions and behaviour of those caring for them. Whatever your views are about the behaviour of those who have contracted AIDS, including those who are homosexuals or drug abusers, your responsibility is to care for all patients without prejudice.

Distressing

Working with a dying person is always distressing. It reminds us of our own mortality, that one day we will ourselves die. It is particularly difficult however, if it is a young child, or someone of our own age or younger who is dying.

In order to protect ourselves from the anxiety and stress which contact with dying causes us, we use a variety of coping tactics, as do the dying person and others close to them. These tactics will be discussed later.

But even in everyday life death and dying is difficult for people to talk about, and the words dying and death are rarely used. Instead we use euphemisms, disguising an unpleasant event with milder words and phrases, such as "he's on the way out; he's slipping away; he won't last much longer; he's snuffed it; he's passed away; she's lost her husband" – you can probably think of others.

Cultural differences

We now live in a multi-cultural society, which means that whatever our own background we are likely to live and work in a community which we share with people who themselves, or whose ancestors, come from many different countries, speak different languages, and have lifestyles, values and beliefs different from our own.

This may mean that, due to their cultural or religious values and beliefs, their attitude to dying and death may be different from our own, which means we have to understand the differences, accept them and respect them. A very useful book on the subject is *Death with dignity* by Jennifer Green[1] which discusses ways of meeting the spiritual needs of patients from different cultural and religious backgrounds.

Choosing for ourselves

Death used to be accepted as the natural conclusion of life, the ultimate experience. Nowadays, however, many of us do resent it. This resentment is well illustrated in the first lines of a poem by Dylan Thomas:

Do not go gentle into that good night
Old age should burn and rave at close of day;
Rage, rage against the dying of the light.

People's reactions to dying and to death vary a lot. It is important that carers do not assume that they know what the dying patient thinks and what they would like to assist them in an appropriate death. They should ask and talk about it. A document relating to patient choice in this area, which has recently appeared in this country, is an *Advance Directive*, or as it is more popularly known, a *Living Will*.

A Living Will is a document which attempts to set out the kind of health care a patient wishes to receive at a time when they are unable to be involved in the actual decision making, for example if they are unconscious, delirious, or otherwise incapacitated. It is an attempt to allow patients the right to refuse treatment in advance, in case they are too ill to choose for themselves, or become unable to express that choice as their condition deteriorates.

A Living Will could also be used to advise those concerned about a person's preference regarding organ donation, instead of or as well as carrying a Donor Card. Just before a patient is expected to die it is difficult to raise the question of organ donation, but if the contents of the Living Will and the existence of a Donor Card are known to the person closest to the patient, the nursing and medical staff, then it is easier to discuss this, indeed the patient may also be involved.

At present Living Wills do not have legal status in this country, but this is currently being discussed by the BMA and the Law Commission.

The dying process

In the late 1960s Dr Elisabeth Kubler-Ross described five stages of dying: *denial, anger, bargaining, depression, acceptance,* which not only patients but also those closest to them, and carers, may experience. Each stage is a way of coping, and care staff need to learn to recognise the stages people are at, and provide the appropriate support.

However what Kubler-Ross does make clear is that people do not go through the stages in a neat sequence but may move backwards and forwards between them, and that the acceptance stage may not be reached at the time of death. Also the patient and those who care about and for them may not experience the same stage at the same time. So care staff have to be very sensitive to what is happening.

Denial

In this stage the patient denies what is happening. He needs support, but care staff should neither encourage nor contradict what he is saying about his illness. This stage gives the patient time to get used to the idea that they are terminally ill, and will die soon.

At this stage the patient or those close to him may try to "shop around", to get another opinion. Staff should realise that this is a normal coping mechanism and should offer people realistic hope, but not lie to them.

Anger

This stage is probably the most difficult for care staff to deal with: the "Why me?" or "Why my baby?" "Why my lover?" "Why my mother?" "It's not fair" stage. The anger may be understandable but the abuse is frequently directed at those closest to the patient, including the carer. During this time those close to the patient and carers feel guilty because they feel helpless and frustrated and this makes them angry as well.

It is important that care staff understand that any abuse and anger is not directed at them personally, but rather at the impending death. All care at this time should be concerned with supporting the dying patient, meeting all their physical needs and maintaining a pleasant attitude – without being too jolly, as this is likely to provoke further anger.

Bargaining

During this stage, which is often quite short, the patient and sometimes those close to him seek ways of postponing the death: "If only I can live long enough to see my grandchild born...If only she can live long enough to see one more Christmas...If only I can go on the holiday we planned...then I'll die happy."

These and other similar remarks are not uncommon, but most common is to try to bargain with God. "If God lets me/my child/my husband/my lover/my mother live I'll be a better person...pray more regularly...go to church..." or something similar. Again the responsibility of care staff is to encourage the patient and others in their realistic hopes, and to make other members of the health care team concerned aware of what has been said. But staff should try to prepare the patient to cope with the disappointment if the bargains, especially those with God, are not apparently kept.

The assistance of the hospital chaplain, or the patient's own priest or minister, may be helpful at this time.

Depression

This may be quite a long stage as the patient, and those close to him, realise that the bargaining has failed, and that the impending death is getting ever closer. Often patients are very quiet during this stage, and just sitting with them and holding their hand is all they need you to do, and the same can be done when close to them visit.

Crying is a healthy sign as this usually shows that the person is coming to accept the closeness of their death. They should not be told off for crying but rather assured that it is okay to cry. They should be comforted while they weep, and there is no shame in staff having a weep along with them. This is a time when the carer should be aware of the patient's spiritual beliefs and needs and make sure they are visited by a priest or representative from their religion if that is important to them.

Acceptance

This is a time of contentment for patients and of sharing with those close to them; a time for tying up loose ends, putting their house in order and saying their farewells. It is often a surprise for those caring for even quite young children who are dying, how quickly they accept the imminence of their death and how practical they are, such as organising what should happen to their favourite toys and their pocket money.

At this time an important part of caring is to make physical contact. Touching is very therapeutic; a simple gesture like holding a patient's hand and stroking their forearm is very comforting.

It is also important to respect the patient's wish to be silent and not to chat, if this is the case. When those close to the patient visit they should also be encouraged to touch and stroke, as it is good for them as well as for the patient. The use of complementary therapies, especially aromatherapy and massage, can be very helpful.

It is important to remember that these stages are *unconscious* coping mechanisms. Not only that, but a patient who is dying does not necessarily go through them in the order set out here, but may move or jump between them. Anger may return at intervals, and some stages may last a lot longer than others.

Finally, it should be remembered that at the time of the death the patient may not have reached the stage of acceptance and neither may some of those who care about him. For all those affected by the death there follows a period of bereavement, which may last up to two years, and they may go through the same stages as experienced during the time before the death as described above.

There are times when staff involved in caring for a patient who is terminally ill may need support, especially when they were close to and fond of the patient.

Sudden death

When the death is sudden and unexpected, then the period immediately following can be very traumatic. Care assistants working in hospital may face extreme reactions of denial and anger by relatives or partner, and this requires the attention of very experienced staff. But an older care assistant with life experience can sometimes be a more suitable person to deal with the situation than a young and inexperienced staff nurse.

Physical care

The main problems when caring for a dying patient are management of pain, control of sickness, care of the skin, control of constipation and respiratory secretions, all of which will cause the patient and visitors distress.

Some of these aspects of physical care are discussed in other chapters, others will be detailed on the patient's care plan. Remember that carrying out activities such as washing, care of the skin, change of position, which must be carried out in private, provide ideal opportunities to talk to the patient, to offer comfort and support, and to find our more about his feelings, hopes and fears. This kind of information should be passed on to the patient's named nurse, or nurse in charge (see *Confidentiality in* Chapter 2).

A lonely experience

Dying can be a very lonely experience, and how we care for somebody who is dying can make this experience better or worse. Many people who are dying feel abandoned; they are physically cut off from those around them, either because they are being nursed in a room on their own, or because they have curtains or screens pulled around their bed, isolating them from the rest of the ward. It could be that the only time they receive attention is when basic activities like feeding or toileting are performed.

Some patients may prefer to be alone; what is important is that the patient is involved in decisions about the care they will receive, rather than routine, ritualistic care dictating what happens and when.

Stress for care staff

Sometimes caring for a dying person causes care staff distress, and there are a variety of tactics we may adopt to help us cope with the stress. These include:

Avoidance: Care staff may avoid going anywhere near the dying person. If contact cannot be avoided, then the staff member does the very least that is necessary when carrying out a task, but ignores the person.

Passing the buck: The care assistant doesn't answer any "awkward" questions, but brushes them aside, by saying things like "You'll have to ask the doctor or the nurse" and at the same time doesn't look at the patient or visitor asking the question. A kinder response would be to say "I don't know but I will ask your nurse to come and speak to you."

Miracle cures: Staff hope that some miracle cure will become available to save the patient's life, perhaps especially if they are young, or when the dying process is going to be prolonged and possibly painful.

Careful conversation: The care assistant avoids asking the sort of questions which would encourage the patient to discuss how they feel about their forthcoming death. For example rather than asking "How are you feeling?" the care assistant says "You're looking better today" or "You're feeling better, aren't you?" then quickly changes the subject before the patient can answer.

Isolation: The dying person may either be nursed in a single room (on occasions this is necessary because of the nature of their illness) or they are hidden from other patients by drawing the curtains. This means visitors are also isolated and care staff are protected from coming into contact with them.

Selective hearing: The carer only hears the most comfortable things the patient says. For example if he says "I'm frightened, the pain is getting worse" then the care assistant will respond to the second part of the statement, perhaps by offering to make enquiries about pain-relieving drugs, and avoid the first part of the statement, the patient's expression of their feelings of fear.

Denial: When talking to the dying patient the care assistant will deny that death is the probable outcome, by saying such things as, "Don't be silly, you're good for another twenty years" or "Don't talk nonsense, whatever gave you that idea?" in response to an awkward question, then continuing the conversation by talking optimistically but unrealistically of the future.

Patient awareness: In some circumstances the care assistant may assume that a patient is unaware of what is going on around them. The care assistant therefore talks freely to a colleague or visitor about the patient and what is wrong with them, or even jokes with a colleague at the patient's expense. Inability to respond does not mean that the patient cannot hear, and even if they cannot, it is still disrespectful to speak in their presence in a way that you would not if they were fully conscious.

It is important to recognise that these tactics are adopted unconsciously; they are the way our minds protect us from a situation that might otherwise be difficult for us to deal with. However, it is vital that these behaviours are recognised and changed, as they prevent us from giving of our best and assisting the patient to an appropriate death.

Training and support

Training courses are available which prepare staff to cope with death and dying, including dealing with awkward questions and difficult moments.

In addition it is useful to hold regular meetings at which issues relating to care of the dying are discussed, or staff support sessions led by a trained counsellor. Such meetings allow staff to discuss their feelings and experiences and to offer each other mutual support and an opportunity to share. Being able to discuss your feelings about death and dying reduces the stress and unhappiness you may experience. (See also Chapter 20, Stress in your life and work.)

Spiritual care

We live in a diverse society and it is essential that carers should be aware of the spiritual beliefs of all those they care for, but especially those who are dying. In particular they need to know what influence the patient's spiritual beliefs may have on their attitude to dying, and what relevance this has on the ritual which has to be observed at the time of death, including rituals such as Last Offices which have to be performed and care of the body (which is important, for example, in the Jewish religion).

A simple solution is to have a set of guidelines and a copy of Jennifer Green's book[1] available on the ward. In addition many religious groups have leaflets to assist care staff, and are always willing to discuss the details with them.

It is also important to remember that some people are atheists or agnostics and their values, beliefs and wishes must also be respected. What would be insulting and disrespectful would be, for example, to ask the hospital chaplain to visit them when they are near to death, because that is what you would want for yourself.

If a funeral service is to be held at a crematorium there is a great deal of freedom for the order of service to be in accordance with the wishes of the person who has died. It may be helpful to the patient if you show that you are aware of this and give them an opportunity to discuss what form of service they would prefer. They should be encouraged to discuss this with the one closest to them if they have not already done so.

Whatever your personal religious beliefs, it is important that you do not impose them on the dying patient, or those close to them, but rather respect their expressed spiritual needs. A mistake at this time could cause the dying person, and those close to them, much distress.

The involvement of a representative of the patient's religion, as soon as they request it, is very important. They then become part of the caring team, offering support to patients, those close to them, and staff.

Close relationship

When a patient is admitted to hospital one of the questions which is asked routinely is the name of the next of kin. For some people, however, their next of kin is not the person who is closest to them – someone else is the most important person in their life. This is the person the dying patient would choose to be with them when they die. This can cause a variety of problems for nursing staff. Some examples are:

• the child whose parents are divorced and who expresses a preference for the parent who does not have custody;

• the teenager who has left home and does not want to see his parents but would prefer his girlfriend or one of his mates to be with him;

• a married person who is having an affair and would prefer the company of the lover;

• a gay or lesbian couple who need to be able to express their affection towards each other just as a heterosexual couple would be able to do;

• a close friend who is more important to the patient than their family, with whom they have lost touch with long ago.

The dilemma for the ward staff is that they are often caught up in the middle of these conflicts. However, at the end of the day it is what the patient wants which is important, and ward staff must make this clear to those "shut out" as gently as possible. Staff must not allow their personal feelings about the rightness of the patient's choice to interfere with their primary function of meeting a patient's needs.

The person closest to the patient should be allowed to be as involved in caring for the patient as is acceptable to them and to the patient, just as the more traditionally recognised family member would be.

However not every patient wants the person closest to them to also function as "nurse." Paul Coffey, who had a heart transplant some years ago and has since died, said that when he was in the Intensive Care Unit his wife, who was a nurse, helped to look after him. But he wanted her to be there as his wife, not as his nurse.

It could be argued that her need was being met, her desire to be involved and do something, but not Paul's which was to have the company of the one he loved. Sometimes there is no conflict between family and the person closest to the patient, in which case all should be involved, with the patient, as part of the caring team.

Whether the one closest to the patient is present when the patient dies depends on a variety of factors. Some may not wish to be there, but will make their goodbyes before they leave the bedside. For others being present will be important. The patient should be allowed to express their own preference; most would prefer not to be alone.

Once this preference is known the ward staff should support both patient and those closest to him in whatever decision they make. If the relative, or person closest to the patient, is not present at the time of death, every effort should be made to ensure that they have the chance to view the body as soon as possible if they so wish, in the company of somebody they know well. At times it may be that care staff and those just bereaved have become close, and it is fine if they want to share their grief with each other, perhaps even crying or praying together.

In conclusion

Death is the inevitable end of life. According to Henry Fielding "It is not death, but dying which is terrible." The responsibility of carers is to ensure that the dying patient's experience is not terrible, but that they experience an "appropriate" death, where they have been involved in the decision making and planning and where their wishes and beliefs are known and respected.

Reference
1. Jennifer Green (1991). Death with Dignity. A *Nursing Times* Publication.

NVQ Value Base Units - Levels 2 & 3
Oa Promote anti-discriminatory practice.
Oc Promote and support individual rights and choice within service delivery.
Od Acknowledge individuals' personal beliefs and identity.
Oe Support individuals through effective communication.

Level 3 Core Units
Z8 Support clients when they are distressed.
Y2 Enable clients to make use of available services and information.

Level 3 Acute Care Endorsement
Z14 Support clients and others at times of loss.

CHAPTER 13

Sexuality and sexual health needs

Lynne Swiatczak and Jim Marr

• Sexuality is vital to the way we feel about ourselves • "Male" and "female" characteristics • The need to be attractive to others • Sexual needs and their expression • Changes and difficulties brought by illness or disability • Don't judge • Simple ways of helping • Sexually transmitted diseases

When we talk about sexuality, most people immediately think of sexual intercourse. The subject of sexuality is, however, much wider than this. A person's sexuality is an expression of their whole identity, personality and relationships with others. Sexuality is about sharing, touching, intimacy and love. It is also about how we feel about ourselves and the effect we have on other people.

Male and female

As we develop from early childhood, we learn about sexuality and how to behave as a boy or a girl. This carries on into adult life, where males are expected to be strong and assertive and to control their feelings, and females to be gentle, caring and sensitive.

However, as we mature we begin to realise that there is a degree of femininity in men and masculinity in women. As people begin to feel more confident and self-aware, they begin to discover themselves and may feel more comfortable in expressing these other aspects. Men begin to realise it is OK to be tender; and women, to be assertive. It is part of our personality.

These feelings vary and may be so strong that they become part of the image a person presents to others. Thus we identify some men as "feminine" and some women as "masculine". Sexuality is expressed in the clothes we wear, the way we behave, our relationships with others, even the music we listen to. It affects all aspects of our lives at work and at leisure.

Sexuality is, therefore, a complex business. It may result in people seeking same-sex relationships in order to fully express themselves and achieve honesty and contentment in their lives. Some may even wish to change their sex completely.

Sexuality is a basic human need (see Maslow's triangle, Chapter 16) and the right of everyone. Because it is so complex, and linked to personal beliefs and values, no one has the right to make judgements about others, providing they are doing no harm to anyone else.

Looking good

When people are ill, often their desire for sexual satisfaction diminishes, but they still retain their need to be attractive to others. So it is important to make sure that hair and skin is kept clean and healthy, that clothing is regularly changed and enhances appearance.

Having their own things around them, using favourite toiletries, jewelry and personal effects – all this helps to maintain individual self-expression and should be encouraged. Being themselves will help them to feel better. Wearing **their own** spectacles, hearing aid or dentures is also very important, especially to elderly people.

Sexual needs

In many caring situations however, people may not feel ill and so their desire for sexual satisfaction remains strong. This can result in feelings which may be expressed negatively as irritability, aggression or emotional upset. Lack of privacy may discourage intimacy with others and aggravate the situation.

It is important, therefore, to be sensitive to needs in these circumstances, and to make time available when patients/clients will be undisturbed and able to relax with visitors.

Sometimes the need to relieve sexual tension finds an outlet in self-stimulation, and care staff should never judge others because their sexual behaviour is not the same as their own. You must be sensitive about this. Erotic stimulation may also be sought through reading materials where no other outlet for sexual activity is available. Remember that these are the patient/client's personal possessions and they should be treated as such. Patients should keep them within their lockers and staff should not remove them. Sexual activity should be expected and treated as normal behaviour.

Well-informed care staff can fulfil a useful role, giving information and guidance if requested, but aware of the sensitivity and embarrassment that may be caused. Sometimes the advice of a more experienced member of staff should be sought.

Sexual health is not only freedom from disease, but is about individual rights and personal fulfilment. Care staff must cultivate a mature non-critical approach in their relationships with others.

Sex and disability

Another aspect of sexuality is the effect of physical health problems on disability. We may immediately think of the woman with a mastectomy but what of the man with a stoma or stroke? There are many problems which affect sexuality in all its forms. An indwelling catheter affects the physical act of sexual intercourse and also affects the way the person feels about themself and their relationships with others.

Sexuality is about how we feel about ourselves, so a physical problem is very likely to cause feelings of fear about intimate relationships with others.

Sometimes patients are admitted to hospital for surgery which will affect their sexuality in the future, and staff caring for the patient must be sensitive to this. Some surgery affects the patient's sexuality in obvious ways, for instance hysterectomy (surgical removal of the womb) or mastectomy (removal of breast). Other forms of surgery can also have similar effects, for example colostomy or amputation. There are also medical conditions which can have the same effects, such as stroke or heart attack. It is therefore important that we do not forget this aspect of care.

Most nurses will include sexuality in their general assessment of the patient on admission and during their stay in hospital. But each patient must be treated as an individual, and this applies especially when deciding whether it is appropriate to assess someone's sexuality. Many people would be horrified if the subject of their sexuality was broached by a stranger during a routine admission. Other patients have a need to discuss this area and would welcome the opportunity.

The care assistant is often the person in whom the patient confides and they must always pass on any important information to the patient's nurse in order that the patient can receive the correct advice. (See the section on *Confidentiality* in Chapter 2.)

Services available

It is not always possible to provide the help patients need while they are in hospital, so discharge planning should take into account any follow-up services the patient may need. Stoma care nurses, breast care nurses and psychologists are but a few of the people available to help patients.

There are other simple ways in which patients can be helped, such as by providing breast prostheses or wigs for patients who have lost their hair through treatments such as chemotherapy for cancer. These measures will only help in part and care staff should not feel that their job is done if they have helped to provide these items.

There is a need for a specialist counselling service for some patients and this must be provided if the patient is to recover fully and take on their former role within society.

Don't judge

The most important thing for all care staff to remember when caring for patients is, **never judge**. The sexual preferences of patients are their own business and each person who has an identified need must be cared for appropriately without prejudice.

Care assistants must remember that they have no right to judge patients and that they must not show any feelings which may hurt or upset the patient. If this is not possible then it is better for the patient to be cared for by another member of staff.

Short term problems

Some of the more usual problems which can occur are short term, associated with a catheter or a wound site. Similar problems are those associated with heart attack. The patient requires correct advice on how and when to resume their sexual activities, and care assistants must either have access to the advice in written form or know which member of staff to refer the patient to.

In the case of catheters the continence adviser can often provide information and advice. Written information is also available.

Patients who have suffered a heart attack or stroke also need information and again this is available in written form. Doctors and nurses usually have this information and can provide advice which is specific to individual patients.

Simple ways of helping

Patients may need what seem to be quite simple measures such as the opportunity to wear make-up and perfume, to dress in their own clothes and to have privacy when partners visit. These things can all be provided without problems, and care assistants must make sure all patients are given this help.

It is also important to treat each patient individually. It is as bad to put make-up on every patient, without choice, than not to provide make-up for anyone! Simple facilities should be available: mirrors, combs, clean personal clothing and hairdressing are just a few examples. In areas where patients stay a short time these things are often not provided, but in longer stay areas for elderly patients, orthopaedic patients or people with mental health problems or learning disabilities, it is important that providing these things should be seen as a basic facility and not as a "perk" or "extra".

Informed choices

All staff should view the patient as a whole person; their sexuality is one part of them which helps to create the whole. For some patients their illness or disability is of long standing and they may feel confident in themselves and their sexuality. This, however, should never be assumed.

Some people may never have received information and advice, and their sex lives may have been inhibited because of this. They may require information and may be angry or depressed that they were not given the right advice in the past.

In these circumstances the care assistant may have to help the patient to accept new information, and may also help the partner by giving them information as requested. But you must make sure that any information you give is up-to-date and accurate, and you must also never "tell" the patient what they should do. Information is given in order for people to make an "informed choice". The choice must be theirs; whatever your own beliefs and values it is not your place to influence that choice.

Sexually transmitted disease

When dealing with sexuality and sexual health needs it is useful also to briefly discuss sexually transmitted diseases. Health care staff work closely with patients often performing quite intimate procedures or sometimes being asked for advise to settle anxieties. It is also important to realise the risk of indirect spread of some of these conditions during caring procedures.

Sometimes these diseases may be spread by indirect means through contact with bedding, towels and clothing or occasionally through direct contact with patients or with their blood or body fluids. It is important therefore to be aware of these risks in order to protect yourself.

This does not mean that you have to cover yourself totally in protective clothing but it does mean always taking simple precautions with every patient, especially when dealing with blood or body fluids such as urine, vomit, faeces, semen and other secretions. This is also important to remember when collecting specimens, cleaning up spillage and disposing of waste products.

Basically there are three main groups of sexually transmitted diseases, those which are spread by:-
1) Parasites 2) Bacteria 3) Viruses

Parasites
These are usually lice or mites which live off the human body either clinging to hair shafts or clothing, or by burrowing under the skin. Although they are mainly spread during intimate or sexual contact, they can be picked up via clothing, bed-clothing or towels and it is not

uncommon for care staff to become infected in this way. Most commonly this group includes Head, Body, Pubic (or Crab) Lice and Scabies.

Bacteria

Diseases spread by bacteria, most commonly during sexual intercourse, include Syphilis and Gonnorhoea

Viruses

Diseases caused by viruses have only come to light in more recent times since technology has advanced enough to detect them. Viruses invade living cells and are thus very difficult to treat without killing off the cells themselves. Throughout the 1980s the Human Immuno-deficiency Virus (HIV) was identified as causing AIDS (Acquired Immune Deficiency Syndrome) and this has been the main focus of health-care since. As yet, there is no known cure for HIV infection and the only means of containing the spread is through public education of precautionary measures.

Everyone is at risk of HIV infection as it is known to spread via blood, body fluids or from mother to child during pregnancy. The misuse of drugs by injection and unprotected sex (during homosexual or heterosexual encounters) has been a major factor in the spread, especially amongst young people.

Accidental transmission via blood or body fluids, has also been reported among health-care workers. Although this risk is small, all care staff are required to be trained, and follow local policies, in order to protect themselves. The main method of preventing spread is through education and sensible precautions which are normally undertaken to prevent cross infection ie wearing gloves for any procedure which involves handling body substances, correct wearing of protective clothing and correct hand washing techniques. (see *Staff hygiene* in Chapter 5).

Points to remember

1. Sexuality is a part of every person.
2. Sexual activity is a "normal" part of human behaviour.
3. Care assistants must not judge patients' sexual behaviour.
4. Sexuality is not just about sexual activity.
4. Make sure any information you give is accurate.
5. Refer patients to other members of staff, such as the stoma care nurse or breast care specialist, as required.
6. Never assume that you know best.
7. Each patient must be allowed to make their own "informed choice".

NVQ Levels 2 & 3 Value Base Units

Oa Promote anti-discriminatory practice.
Ob Maintain confidentiality of information.
Oc Promote and support individual rights and choice within service delivery.
Od Acknowledge individuals' personal beliefs and identity.
Oe Support individuals through effective communication.

Levels 2 & 3 Core Units

U4 Contribute to the health, safety and security of individuals and their environment.
U5 Obtain, transmit and store information relating to the delivery of a care service.

Level 3 Core Unit

Y2 Enable clients to make use of available services and information.

Level 2 Direct Care Endorsement

Z9 Enable clients to maintain their personal hygiene and appearance.

CHAPTER 14

Caring for adults in medical and surgical wards

Anne Eaton

• Welcoming new patients • Your role in the admission procedure • The patient admitted in an emergency • Medical care • Surgery: tests and investigations, preparing the patient • After the operation: observations and care • The gynaecology patient

As a care assistant in medicine, surgery and gynaecology, you will meet and care for patients of all ages, with different ethnic and religious backgrounds and with many and varied medical conditions. You will care for these patients from admission to discharge (or a peaceful death). This chapter aims to describe your role as a member of the ward team.

Admission to hospital

Admission to hospital, whether to a medical, surgical or gynaecology ward, is a very worrying experience for anyone. From the patient's point of view, no condition or potential surgery is "minor" (though the medical and nursing staff may call it that) and the care assistant should take this into account at all times, treating every patient as an individual.

The care assistant may be one of the first members of staff to greet new patients and their relatives, and first impressions do count for a great deal. Be welcoming to new patients and let them know that they are expected, even if their admission is an emergency.

Preparation

Before the expected admission, it is necessary to prepare the bed and surrounding area, and make sure the locker is empty and clean. It is also necessary to prepare beforehand any forms and documents which may be needed – for example temperature, pulse, respiration and blood pressure charts, fluid balance charts, nursing records and so on – so that the new admission is given your full attention on arrival. All this preparation may be carried out under the supervision of the trained nurse.

On arrival

When new patients arrive, it is important to greet them by name, introduce yourself and escort them to their bed. If possible, it is advisable to leave them alone to undress (if indeed they need to undress at this point). This is especially relevant when a new patient is admitted as non-emergency to a surgical or to a gynaecology ward. Alternatively, help with undressing may be necessary.

Charts and records

During the admission procedure, you may be working independently or with a qualified nurse, depending upon the patient's condition and needs. A lot of information will be obtained at this time and it is important to write down and report all findings, even if you think they are not important. Each hospital will have its own policy about the care assistant's role in filling in charts and records.

The ward and its routine

New patients need help to get used to their new environment. If their condition allows, they should be given a tour of the ward. In particular, showing them the toilet and bathroom areas, their immediate bed area and introducing them to their new "neighbours" may play a part in alleviating anxiety at this time.

Most patients will appreciate being given some idea of the day-to-day routine – meal times, visiting times, access to the patients' telephone – and having their questions answered truthfully and promptly. If you are not able to answer any questions, then you must immediately refer them to the nurse in charge of the patient's care.

Identification

All admissions to hospital, emergency and non-emergency, will be fitted with an identification bracelet, stating their name, date of birth, ward, consultant and record number. This is vital in case the patient's condition alters and he cannot tell you his name, for example if he becomes unconscious or confused.

Confidentiality

Keeping information about patients confidential is a vital aspect of the care assistant's role, and confidentiality must be respected at all times. However, if a patient gives you information that will affect their care, then your responsibility is to explain to the patient that you must pass on this information to the nurse in charge of their care.

The emergency admission

Some patients are admitted because their condition needs immediate attention. They will have been referred as an emergency by their own general practitioner, or through the accident and emergency department.

This is an extremely anxious time for all concerned, and although the qualified nurse will be the key person in the admission procedure, your role is very important, both in the pre-admission preparation and as an assistant to the nurse in the immediate admission phase.

Relatives or friends may have accompanied the patient into hospital and they will also be in need of advice and support at this worrying time. The care assistant will probably be asked to look after the visitors. Greet them with a friendly word and explanation if needed; this will promote confidence and contribute to relieving anxiety, as well as help to establish good relationships.

Tests and investigations

A new patient may have to undergo many different investigations and tests. Some of these are within the role of the care assistant – taking and recording blood pressure and temperature, testing urine, and so on. It is vital that you understand the principles related to these tests, how to perform them, how to distinguish between normal and abnormal and how to record and report all findings in the right place and to the appropriate person. Each hospital has its own policy regarding the role of the care assistant in investigations.

Other procedures are carried out by a qualified nurse or doctor, but you are likely to assist them in undertaking such procedures as venepuncture, lumbar puncture and vaginal examination.

For these procedures you may need to be able to prepare the necessary equipment, prepare the patient or environment, support the patient and answer questions, if possible, after the procedure has been explained to them by the professional. You may be able to assist the professional during the procedure, assist in monitoring the patient afterwards, and help to clear away the equipment, returning the environment to normal.

Scanning and x-rays

Some investigations cannot be undertaken on the ward, because specialised equipment is used. These investigations, such as ultra-sound scan, barium meal and chest x-ray, will aid the doctor in making the correct diagnosis and prescribing appropriate treatment.

For most investigations, special preparation is needed. It is vital that the patient and all care staff are aware of exactly what preparation is required, so that instructions can be carried out exactly – otherwise the investigation might have to be repeated.

If the patient's condition allows, you might be the person who escorts them to the relevant department, or even a different hospital. Good communication skills are necessary here (see Chapter 3), as well as knowledge of the patient and their condition. You will be meeting and

working with many different staff, for example ambulance personnel, radiographers or consultant doctors, and your contribution will play a vital part in the procedure and its outcome.

Preparation for surgery

Patients admitted for a surgical operation will either be admitted from a waiting list or as an emergency.

Most **non-emergency** patients will be admitted the day before their operation. Any necessary investigations will be performed in this time. Most surgical patients also need to have the operation site shaved in order to help prevent a wound infection after the operation. Not all operations require shaving however.

All patients will need to sign a form giving their **consent** for the operation to be performed. This is the responsibility of the doctor, but the patient may ask the care assistant questions about it, which must be answered by the appropriate person, usually the nurse in charge of the patient's care.

The patient must **not eat or drink** for at least four hours before the operation. This is so that the stomach will be empty, which will reduce the risk of complications from vomiting during and after surgery. (Because they are unconscious they may inhale the vomit into their lungs and either block the airway or cause serious infection).

You will need to tell the patient the important reasons why they must not eat, so that they will co-operate with your instructions. Also a "Nil by mouth" sign will be placed on the patient's bed, to inform all staff and visitors.

Personal hygiene needs to be attended to immediately before surgery. If the patient is to have their surgery in the morning, they may be encouraged to have a **bath or shower** during breakfast time, in order to avoid food! A clean theatre gown must then be worn and the patient advised to rest in their clean bed.

The **site of the operation** may have been marked by the surgeon – left leg, right breast, for example – and it is important that the patient or care assistant does not wash away this identification.

The patient needs lots of **reassurance** at this time; this must be given and any questions answered by the appropriate person. It has been proved that information about care can improve and speed up the post-operative recovery of the patient.

Special procedures may be performed before surgery, for example insertion of an intravenous infusion or urinary catheter, and you may assist in the performance of these procedures.

Patients may be prescribed some **medication**, usually given as an intra-muscular injection by the qualified nurse just before the time of the operation. This medication (called the "pre-med") will help the patient relax, so the environment needs to be kept as quiet as possible to allow them to rest. After this the patient will be called for and transferred to the operating department, accompanied by a qualified nurse.

While the patient is away from the ward their **bed area must be prepared** for their return. Any equipment which will be needed must be collected and appropriately positioned. For example, an infusion stand is often needed.

After the operation

On arrival back at the ward the patient will be conscious but sleepy, and the qualified nurse will be very involved in the immediate post-operative period, with your assistance.

Observations of blood pressure, pulse rate, respiratory (breathing) rate, level of consciousness, skin colour, pain, wound site and drainage, and urine output will be undertaken frequently, usually half-hourly. As the patient's condition improves and becomes stable, some of these observations may be delegated to you. Careful measurement, recording and reporting of these observations is vital for the detection of post-operative complications.

SIGNS OF PAIN AND DISTRESS

- **Facial expression – frown/grimace**
- **Body position - protecting or "guarding" the painful area**
- **Raised respiratory (breathing) rate**
- **Raised pulse rate**
- **Withdrawal and unwillingness to communicate with staff or other patients**
- **Frequent requests for medication to relieve pain**
- **Anger**
- **Tears**
- **Restlessness**

The patient must be **kept pain-free** at all times and you will need to be aware of verbal and non-verbal signs that the patient is distressed (see list above). The care assistant must be alert to these signs at all times and they should be reported to the nurse or doctor without delay. Reassurance in the form of hand-holding, talking and simply being there will be vital aspects of care that the patient will need, and which you can deliver. A pain-free post-operative period enables the patient to recover more quickly.

As the patient's post-operative condition improves, then you will **assist them to wash** and put on their own night clothes.

Before **oral fluid and/or food** is given,

the care assistant must check the care plan and consult the nurse in charge of the patient's care. When they will be allowed to eat and drink very much depends upon their surgery, condition and current progress.

When diet and fluids are allowed, they are given in small amounts and slowly, and their effects on the patient observed and monitored closely. Any adverse symptoms, such as vomiting, must be reported immediately.

Most patients recover relatively quickly from surgery, and you must gently encourage them to regain independence in preparation for discharge.

Emergency surgery

The condition of some patients is such that they need urgent surgery for potentially life-threatening conditions.

Most of the areas already covered will also apply to the emergency admission, but the speed at which these procedures are undertaken is usually much faster. The care assistant will, in these situations, assist the qualified staff in the smooth admission, preparation, and transfer to the operating department of the acutely ill patient. Your skills in communicating with both patients and their families are vital here.

Medical care

Patients admitted to a medical ward may be suffering from any one of a multitude of conditions. On most medical wards, the care assistant will look after patients with chest conditions, heart conditions, circulatory problems and blood disorders.

Medicine is like a large jigsaw puzzle: the entire care team gathers clues relating to the patient's signs and symptoms, and the pieces are put together until a picture emerges which aids the doctor in the diagnosis of the patient's condition.

The care assistant is a member of this team, and what may seem trivial tasks, such as urine testing, may be vital in the correct diagnosis and subsequent treatment of the medical patient. No information should be judged as irrelevant; it should always be passed on to the appropriate member of the care team.

Encouraging independence
Patients should be encouraged to remain as independent as possible in the areas of personal hygiene, mobility and nutrition. For many patients, some independence will be lost, and patience and tact must be exercised in order to care for the patient who may well feel frustrated and angry in the loss of independence, for example the patient who has had a cerebrovascular accident (stroke).

An awareness of the patient's physical and psychological condition will be helpful in understanding care and giving the best care possible. Basic care skills, covered in other chapters, are vital in caring for all patients, and the care assistant's role in the medical ward is of major importance.

The gynaecology patient

The care already described applies also to patients admitted to the gynaecology ward, but there are some special aspects of care to take into account when caring for women undergoing gynaecological surgery.

Many aspects of a woman's personal life may need to be investigated and assessed because they relate to her specific gynaecological condition. The care assistant needs to respect the patient's confidentiality and not discuss any details of care with anyone, not even the patient's partner, but refer all enquiries to the nurse in charge of the patient's care. Patients may have complicated personal lives and it is not your place to judge, it is your place to care.

You may find yourself in an ethical dilemma when working on a gynaecology ward, and any feelings of conflict should be discussed, in private, with the nurse in charge. Conflict may arise, for example, when caring for a woman undergoing termination of pregnancy.

Nevertheless, your role is to deliver care in a totally non-discriminatory manner to all patients. Tact and diplomacy, as well as compassion and empathy, are vital components in care delivery.

Conclusion

For the care assistant employed in acute medicine, surgery or gynaecology, life is never dull! The work is always full and varied and the patients offer a challenge to any care giver. Job satisfaction can be limitless in these situations and the care assistant can gain competence day by day in new knowledge and skills.

Points to remember

1. The care assistant will play a vital part in care.
2. Remember to treat all patients as individuals with different abilities and needs.
3. Report and record all findings to the appropriate person and in the appropriate place, in order that no information is lost.
4. Communication skills (see Chapter 3) are vital in this work.
5. Your observational skills also play a major part in the ongoing care of your patients.

NVQ Levels 2 & 3 Value Base Units:
Oa. Promote indiscriminatory factors.
Ob. Maintain confidentiality of information.
Oc. Promote and support individual rights and choice within service delivery.
Oe. Support individuals through effective communication.

Level 2 Core Units
W2 Contribute to the ongoing support of clients and others significant to them.
W3. Support clients in transition due to their care requirements.

Levels 2 & 3 Core Unit
U5 Obtain, transmit and store information relating to the delivery of a care service.

Level 3 Core Unit
Z8 Support clients when they are distressed.

Level 2 Direct Care Endorsement
Z9 Enable clients to maintain their personal hygiene and appearance.
Z19 Enable clients to achieve physical comfort.

Level 3 Acute Care Endorsement
X12 Support professionals with clinical activities.
X19 Prepare and undertake agreed ongoing clinical activities with clients in acute care settings.
U3 Prepare and maintain environments for clinical procedures.

CHAPTER 15

Critical care and emergencies

Lynn Sbaih

• Your role in an emergency – life support and first aid • Machines and information technology • Working as a team with qualified staff • The "buddy" system of providing care

Critical care areas in the hospital where care assistants may work include:

• Accident and emergency department (A/E)
• Intensive care unit (ITU)
• Operating theatre/room
• Renal unit
• Coronary care unit

All these areas cater for both children and adults, including elderly people. The critical care area may be large or small in size and in the number of patients received. Areas such as A/E and ITU receive people with a wide range of injuries and illness, acute or chronic. The operating theatre caters for people requiring surgery, the renal unit for persons with specific problems relating to the kidneys, and the coronary care unit for people with acute heart problems.

Emergencies

Sudden emergencies occur in these critical areas, and care assistants need to be aware of what they should do during an emergency. Although you will never be expected to look after the patient by yourself, it will help you to know that most emergencies relate to problems with airway, breathing and circulation.

Before starting work in a critical care area all care assistants should have received training and be competent in basic life support and first aid measures, including

- knowing when and how to call for help
- positioning the patient
- performing rescue breathing
- dealing with other breathing problems
- performing external chest compression
- dealing with choking
- dealing with fainting
- dealing with bleeding.

Competence in these skills will enable you to assist the qualified nurse during an emergency. The type and frequency of emergencies will vary depending on the area in which you work. For example in the A/E department the care assistant will witness bleeding and fainting as well as patients who have stopped breathing and require the support of drugs and machines. In the ITU and operating

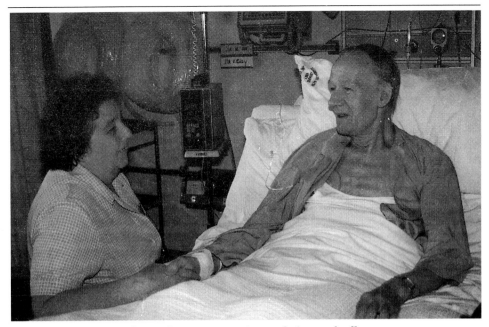

The care assistant can offer much support to patients, relatives and colleagues.

theatre the care assistant is more likely to be involved in emergencies associated with the patient stopping breathing.

Key points
• Emergencies can happen without warning, so you must be prepared for an emergency at all times. You will be involved in ensuring that the critical care environment is safe at all times and that machinery is checked and in full working order.
• Qualified nurses in the critical care area are trained to deal with all emergencies, and they will support you during an emergency.
• The care assistant can offer much support to patients, relatives and colleagues. What support you can give needs to be discussed with qualified nurses before the emergency occurs.
• Following an emergency situation all staff involved, including care assistants, should discuss what happened and offer suggestions for better management of similar situations in future.

Machines

The care assistant needs to become familiar with any machines used in their work area. You will not be expected to use machines unsupervised, but to assist in their use, maintenance and checking under the supervision of a qualified nurse.

Key points
• Get to know how machines work but remember that the use of machines remains the responsibility of the qualified nurse and/or doctor.

Information technology

Many areas have computer terminals to assist qualified nurses in the documentation of care assessment, planning, implementation and evaluation. Again the care assistant will not be expected to record information unless under the supervision of a qualified nurse.

Key point
• Get to know how information technology is used in your area.

Teamwork

Care assistants are required to work very closely with other members of the critical care team. Members of this team may include:
- qualified nurses
- care assistants
- doctors
- physiotherapists
- occupational therapists
- operating department assistants.

Key points
• Get to know the routine of nurses in your area, including how they plan their day.
• Get to know how nurses deal with sudden change in your area.
• Get to know the members of the critical care team.

Providing care

Qualified nurses in critical care areas are responsible for assessing, planning, implementing and evaluating patient and family care. The care assistant can contribute in a number of ways:

- helping to make patients comfortable

- helping to turn patients

- helping to feed patients and their families

- talking and listening to patients and their families

- providing company for the patient and their family.

One way in which the care assistant can assist the nurse in the critical care area is through a "buddy" system.

The "buddy" system
Working together as "buddies" allows

THE "BUDDY" SYSTEM
• The qualified nurse and care assistant will work as a team to provide care for the patient and family.

• All opportunities will be taken to ensure the patient and family are able to choose to be involved in their own care, and do become involved in their own care.

• The care provided will aim to meet all the needs and requirements of the patient and family.

• The qualified nurse will aim to encourage the care assistant to develop knowledge and skills to allow continuation of assistance in the care delivery plan.

• The care assistant will aim to encourage the qualified nurse to develop knowledge and skills to maintain a high standard of care to the patient and family.

• The qualified nurse and care assistant remain accountable for the decisions they make and the care they give to the patient and family.

Example of an agreed information poster about the critical care "buddy" system.

both the care assistant and the qualified nurse to develop a team approach to the care of the person and family. It also allows the care assistant to develop skills and knowledge related to looking after people in the critical care area. Together you and the qualified nurse can provide a wider range of services to the patient and family.

For the buddy system to work, care assistants need to become familiar with the way nurses provide care in the critical care area. Everyone involved needs to meet and discuss regularly how the system should work, and come to an agreement on what care can be provided by whom and how. Then the agreed information can be put on a poster (see example, right) to remind everyone of the aims of the buddy system.

Key points
• It is important that all nurses, qualified and unqualified, are involved in this approach to the planning of work, otherwise true partnership will not take place.
• The care assistant can positively contribute to care delivery within the clinical area. Skills and knowledge can be exchanged and developed by taking part in regular discussion with qualified nurses.

Different needs

You will find that the changing needs of patients and their families in the critical care area will determine how skills and knowledge are developed. For example in the A/E department you will develop skills in assisting the qualified nurses in making sure patients have sufficient to eat and drink. In the ITU this may be difficult as most patients are not able to eat or drink normally. You may therefore find you develop skills and knowledge in providing food and drink for the relatives of patients.

In conclusion, the aim of the care assistant is to provide care under supervision for patients in the critical care area. Care has to be continuous and supervised by a qualified nurse.

Points to remember

1. The care assistant should take an active part in the planning and delivery of care to meet changing patient and family priorities in the critical care area, under the supervision of the qualified nurse.

2. You should be aware of your role in an emergency and the support required by other colleagues, patients and their families.

3. You should work with other members of the critical care team and help formulate statements which illustrate how care is delivered in partnership with qualified nurses in the critical care area.

4. You should be aware of machines used in the area and contribute to the care and maintenance of these machines.

5. You should be familiar with the use of information technology in your work area.

6. You should be aware of the movement of patients in your work area and be aware of how the transfer of patients is planned and undertaken, under the supervision of a qualified nurse.

Resources
Gee K (1993) *Cardiopulmonary resuscitation: basic life support skills: 2.* British Journal of Nursing Vol 2 No 2 p138-141.

NVQ Levels 2 & 3 Core Units
U4 Contribute to the health, safety and security of individuals and their care environment.
U5 Obtain, transmit and store information relating to the delivery of a care service.

Level 2 Core Unit
W2 Contribute to the ongoing support of clients and other significant to them.
W3 Support clients in transition due to their care requirements.

CHAPTER 16

Caring for older people

James Marr

• Quality of life and individual choice • Older people still feel young inside • From basic needs to things that make life worth living • Physical, mental and social health in old age • Your attitude and commitment to a high standard of care

Caring for older people is a complex but very rewarding part of the modern healthcare system. It is often described as "basic" care by those who do not properly understand it, or those who work in areas which do not have enough resources to give care at a high enough level to meet all the needs of their patients or clients.

Enjoying life

Like other age groups, the quality of older people's lives is based on "feeling good" and enjoying the good things in life. This enjoyment may come from a whole range of activities and experiences which we value as individuals and which make us different from our friends.

If everyone liked to do the same things every day, life would be very dull and boring and we would soon become fed up and lose interest. Similarly, each of us has ideas about what we want from our lives and what we feel is important to us. No one has the right to make up our minds for us, or to make decisions on our behalf without asking us.

These feelings that we have about ourselves do not age. As people get older, they still "feel" young inside. Ask older people what age they "feel" they are, and you will be surprised at what they say.

It is important therefore, when caring for older people, to find out about them as individuals – what they have done in their lives and the things that are important to them. In this way we gain some understanding of "what makes them tick" and this helps us to decide, with them, what care they require and how we can continue to help them make life interesting. These are the things that we all value, and which add stimulation and quality to our lives. Our hopes, dreams and ambitions keep us "motivated".

About fifty years ago, an American psychologist called Abraham Maslow, described this "motivation" and illustrated it as a triangle which he divided into five sections (see Fig. 1 opposite).

At the bottom of the triangle are the things in life which are very basic for survival but, as we move up the triangle,

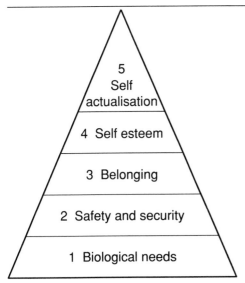

Fig. 1: Maslow's triangle or "hierarchy" of human needs.

we identify other factors which add quality, interest and meaning to life. These factors are described as our "needs" and, according to Maslow, are laid out in order of importance to us as human beings.

The sections are more clearly described in this way:

1. Biological needs

These are the very basic things which we need to keep us alive such as air, water, food, shelter, comfort, rest and sleep, and sex.

2. Safety and security

This is about having a safe place to stay with no worries about money or legal problems. It is also about being able to make full use of our senses such as sight, hearing, touch, taste and smell.

3. Belonging

This section deals with our close relationships with others – friends, family, carers and pets – who "mean" something and who make up our "social" lives.

4. Self esteem

At this level we need to feel "useful" and "in control" of our lives and to be important to, or "needed" by, others. These are feelings of contentment and satisfaction.

5. Self-actualisation

This is the most complex section and involves our personal philosophy of life – what life means to us. At this level there is a need for self-expression and creativity, to enjoy things which we see as worthwhile, good and beautiful. This may involve stimulation and appreciation of music or art, or may be spiritual awareness, or the preparation for a meaningful death.

According to Maslow, to gain full satisfaction and contentment in life, each human being strives to "move up" the triangle, meeting the "needs" described in each section before they can progress. In this way, quality of life is improved and increasing fulfilment is gained. A life striving each day to achieve only the bare necessities at the bottom of the triangle is only an existence and may truly be described as "basic".

This triangle, or model, is useful when caring for older people because it helps care staff to view them as individuals and helps to challenge ideas about the level of care which is given.

Sometimes care is based around "activities of living" which are the basic tasks (such as washing and dressing) we all perform every day, but try to complete as quickly as possible so that time is spent on the things we enjoy.

If care only involves meeting these very basic needs then it will be dull and boring, not only for patients, but also for the care staff themselves. When "care" is based at such a low level, then it may indeed be described as basic and it is not what true caring involves. Older people need to be "cared about" as much as "cared for". It is important, therefore, to plan care with your patient, and to review it regularly as needs are constantly changing (see *Nursing care plan* on p.37).

The ageing process

In modern society, a huge industry has developed with products designed to keep us looking younger and staying fitter. Youthfulness has not only to be gained, but also maintained. Unfortunately this means that ageing is viewed less positively and is often seen as a "problem". Negative attitudes may therefore develop, which care staff may bring to their work with older patients.

When people are described as "old" or "elderly", this usually means they have reached the age of retirement, which is around 65 years. Most people at this age however, do not think of themselves as old. "Old age" is usually thought to involve some degree of ill-health or disability. In healthcare settings catering for older people, therefore, there may be a very wide range of ages (from sixties to over 100) and a wide range of ability and independence. This is another good reason why care must be given on an individual basis.

Physical health

Most older people are relatively healthy and age has little to do with health. Many young people suffer from poor health, but on the other hand, many old people enjoy good health. Human potential, therefore, is not related to age. As we develop from infancy, our skills and abilities change during the course of our lives, and so old age is a further stage of this normal development process.

Unfortunately, as we grow older, our bodies (like machines) may not function as well, and we may become "less able" than before. At this stage it may take more time or effort to do things, though it does not mean that the person is "ill". The abilities of older people, therefore, will range according to their health: from *normal* to *less able* to *ill health*.

At different stages they will need different levels of help, and it is good to encourage them to do as much for themselves as they can. Because of the changes which occur with ageing, care planned for many older people may be focused on common problems such as mobility, continence, communication and maintaining independence.

Illnesses which affect older people are the same as those affecting younger age groups but increased ageing lowers resistance and older people tend to become more ill more quickly.

Sometimes people experience a variety of ailments as they go through life, and when they eventually need care it appears more complicated because of the different treatments for the different ailments. Often they will be prescribed a number of medications, and the effects of these may need to be balanced carefully with each other. It is important therefore, to report any problems which may arise, as it may mean that these prescriptions need to be altered.

Mental health

Just as happens with younger people, the stresses and strains of everyday life may affect the mental health of our elders. Most of us experience "good" and "bad" days when our mood alters accordingly, and these feelings are the same in older people.

As we mature, we learn to cope with these negative feelings and try not to let them affect other people. Sometimes, however, these coping strategies may not work and our mental health may be affected.

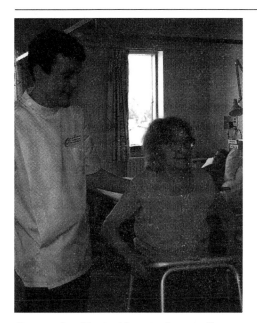

It may take older people more time or effort to to things, but that does not mean they are ill.

Older people often experience a variety of negative events in their lives, such as illness, bereavement or poverty, which cause them to become isolated from others. Often they become lonely and depressed and may need help to cope with their feelings and gain some quality in their lives.

Another common mental health issue of older people is **confusion**. Sometimes confusion may be the first sign of a physical illness and may develop over a very short period of time. However, sometimes it is a sign of a more serious mental health problem called **dementia**. This condition is caused by brain cells dying off much more rapidly than they should, and so the sufferer gradually begins to lose all the things that they have learned throughout their lives. It is a distressing condition for the patient and also for their family and friends.

Whichever type of confusion is present, the older person needs help to make sense of their surroundings by being gently reminded of the information which they are unable to recall. Sometimes they may also display unusual behaviour which may be similarly managed with sympathetic handling.

Social health

After the age of retirement, many older people begin to feel a loss of purpose in their lives. Previously they may have led very busy active lives, working, raising a family and running a home. At this stage they may feel that time is heavy on their hands, and they are "not needed".

Sometimes this may cause them to withdraw from their social activities which further increases their loss. It is important, therefore, to encourage older people to remain active and involved with others as this in turn gives meaning and quality to their lives. With increasing age this activity may have to be reduced but energies may be channelled into other worthwhile causes, such as using handicraft skills for charity or fundraising. In this way a sense of purpose is maintained and encouraged.

Standards of care

Older people deserve to be "cared about", not just "cared for". This means that those involved in their care must have a positive attitude towards them and be committed to giving them the same standard of care they would wish their own grandparents, parents or themselves to have. A good self-check therefore is to occasionally ask "is this the way I would like my grandmother/father, or myself, to be treated ?"

Caring for older people is hard work, both physically and emotionally, and it is important to talk to someone if you are feeling stressed. It is unfair, and bad practice, to deliver a poor standard of care because you are "tired out".

Older people are individuals and have a right to be treated with respect and dignity in an environment which is suited to their special needs. They have the right to choose and make decisions about their care and how and where they should live. Your role is to help them to make these choices and decisions in the care which you plan *with* them.

Remember the stages in Maslow's triangle and help your patients to reach as high as they can.

Points to remember

1. All older people are different and the care given should be different for each one in order to meet their individual needs.
2. It is not enough to provide only "basic" care as that does not enhance the quality of their lives. Higher needs should also be met.
3. Older people suffer from the same types of illnesses as younger age groups but the process of ageing may complicate these or the treatment of them.
4. Throughout their care, older people should be encouraged to be as independent as possible, and to have as much power, information and choice to enable them to make decisions and plans about their own lives.

NVQ Levels 2 & 3 Value Base Units
Oc Promote and support individual rights and choice within service delivery.
Od Acknowledge individuals' personal beliefs and identity.

Level 2 Core Unit
W2 Contribute to the ongoing support of clients and others significant to them.

CHAPTER 17

Caring for people with mental health difficulties

Tim Martin

• A different, rewarding role for the care assistant • The skills you need – perception, communication, observation • How to build up a helpful, therapeutic relationship • Sharing information • Working as a team • Wider responsibilities

Caring for individuals suffering from mental health difficulties can be an absorbing and rewarding area in which to work. One of its most interesting aspects is its "mystery". Mystery because unlike most other scientific pursuits it deals with often unseen, unmeasurable and inexplicable phenomena. Unlike medicine or surgery, there is no broken leg that can be felt, set and plastered; no bloody wounds to be cleaned and stitched; no tumours that can be scanned and surgically removed.

Popular public perceptions of mental health care are often gained from films such as *One Flew Over The Cuckoo's Nest* or *Silence of the Lambs,* where workers only leave the protection of offices to tighten the buckles of straitjackets on dangerous aggressive patients.

This notion was and is still reinforced by the older mental asylums which were built away from communities, and hidden behind walls. Fortunately such images of mental health care bear no resemblance to present-day reality.

People suffering with mental health difficulties may appear to be very ordinary and act in a very normal way, particularly to the inexperienced eye. Discovering each individual's particular needs and responding to them with warmth and understanding, is the challenge for care staff.

Learning to cope with life

Each of us is a unique individual, genetically produced by parents, developed through a unique series of life experiences, and living in a unique life situation. So each of us reacts uniquely to the difficulties life inevitably brings.

Most of us are fortunate: we have the capacity to learn to cope with many difficult situations, and move successfully through life. The broadest definition of a person with mental health difficulties could be, an individual who fails to cope with their life situation.

Your role

Stigma and public ignorance lead many people to believe mental illness is inevitably dangerous and incurable, and that society should be protected from mentally ill people. The mental health care worker's true role may not be obvious to an outsider; the image of the jailer armed with powerful medication is a difficult one to dispel.

Your role in reality is much less sensational. In order to help someone, you must first begin to understand them as an individual, and learn the nature of their difficulties.

Without the luxury of visible signs and symptoms or advanced technology to investigate and monitor mental health needs, members of the caring team have to rely on their own personal skills to gain the essential information. These vital skills are described under the headings that follow.

Perception

Perception is a key part of our lives. We are constantly receiving information through our senses, and taking action based on this information. Often this "data-analysis" is done so often we are not consciously aware we are doing it. How many times have you completed a task or activity, then when you stop and think back, you cannot remember the details of the task – it has become automatic.

To collect and interpret information from clients, it is important to be very aware of your perceptions. Seemingly unimportant remarks or changes in behaviour or appearance can give clues to an individual's difficulties and needs.

And of course this is a two way process. It is just as important for you to be aware of how you are perceived by others. Clients are just as capable of picking up clues about our thoughts. It is impossible for us to like or relate well to everyone!

Communication

Communication is the most important component of mental health care. Your aim is to understand the individual, and effective communication with them is the best way to achieve that understanding.

Verbal communication

Talking and asking questions is the most obvious method of finding things out, but it takes thought and practice to be effective.

Apart from considering the content of a conversation, we must also learn to understand other verbal cues such as the tone of voice, volume and word emphasis – all of which help to build up the true meaning of what is being said.

We may say one thing, while meaning or thinking something completely different. This can be either intentional or unconscious, but by carefully listening to the *way* things are said as well as *what* is said, we can learn much.

Non-verbal communication

Your understanding and awareness of the ways people communicate without words, is crucial. For example, eye contact is central to conversation: avoiding eye contact suggests mistrust, but too much can be threatening. Eye level is also important: physically looking up to someone can feel threatening (to you), looking down on someone can suggest dominance. Try to position yourself so that your eyes are on a level with those of the person with whom you are talking.

Observation

Aspects of an individual's behaviour give the observer vital clues to their inner thoughts and feelings, that may in turn be essential to understanding their difficulties or successfully delivering care.

Position: This may tell us a good deal. Is the person choosing to distance themself from others, sitting away in a corner? Perhaps they are feeling low or unworthy? Conversely, are they invading others' personal space, looming over them? Perhaps they are angry or frustrated ?

Posture: A "closed" posture, for example sitting facing away from others with arms and legs crossed, suggests a disinterest in or fear of communication. Whereas sitting facing someone with arms and legs uncrossed may suggest a willingness for approach or involvement.

Appearance: We automatically infer a lot of information from the way a person looks, and this can influence what we expect of them and how we behave towards them if we are not careful. We might assume, for instance, that someone who is scruffy or dishevelled would lack motivation in other aspects of their life, whereas someone in a smart suit might be assumed competent and efficient. Both assumptions could be hopelessly inaccurate and misleading.

Interaction with environment: The way a person behaves in their environment gives clues. Someone smashing window panes is obviously disturbed with problems that need addressing immediately. But a different individual who sits staring at the wall may have equally pressing needs.

The above pointers are given as examples for guidance only. Each individual is unique, so to have any meaning an observation must be made and considered in context. A certain amount of knowledge and under-standing of the individual is essential in order to judge what significance the observed activity has for them.

Rapport

To begin to build a helpful, therapeutic relationship with the client, the care assistant has to put all the above techniques into practice and work towards a mutual understanding, or "rapport". This is essential if you are to help them, because not many people are willing to share their difficulties with someone they consider to be a stranger.

You must be patient in your attempt to build a rapport. Remember that the client's situation and condition may well make them feel threatened and mistrustful of others. Try to "read" the situation and non-verbal clues to choose the best times to approach the client, and "read" the client's reactions to evaluate whether they are open and receptive to your efforts. If the client is becoming hostile or angry for instance, might it be better to withdraw and try again at another time?

In conversation it is better to have an honest open approach to the client. Showing the client that you have *empathy* toward them is important. Empathy means showing you care about how they feel, and are willing to try to understand their situation, rather than *sympathy* which may be seen as condescending.

Be reliable

Being reliable is very important. It is very easy to promise to do something for a client, particularly if you are busy at the time, and because you might have a further twenty clients to think about, you forget to do it. The client however might have nothing else to think about but your promise, which could become very significant to them as a consequence.

A little thing (to you) such as taking someone to the shop at a certain time, might become central to their day. Failure to be reliable could have severe repercussions on your relationship. Don't make promises you might not be able to keep.

Professional boundaries

A successful rapport can often be a difficult balance to achieve. Your role is to get to know the person, develop an understanding and empathy for them, allow them to begin to know and trust you, and offer your services as a non-judgemental "friend". All this while always maintaining a professional overview of the relationship and situation.

Confidentiality of information is important, but care must be taken to acknowledge the boundaries within which you are working. It is important that you share information with other care workers, for the client's benefit in terms of consistency and continuity, and for your own benefit to ensure that you have the support and supervision of others and maintain a balanced perspective of the situation. Over-involvement and lack of supervision and support can be damaging to all concerned.

Sharing information

An important part of building rapport is developing trust. You should always endeavour to keep the client informed of what is happening to and around them. This means taking the time to explain actions and procedures to them in language they can understand, and encouraging their questioning and involvement in their own care process.

Remember you are likely to be the main contact between the client and the care system, so the client may ask you anything. It is important that you make sure you *can* answer the question before you try. Details of their illness or treatment for example are better explained by a qualified nurse or doctor. In some rare instances there may be information that the client should not be told (for example the telephone number of relatives). The golden rule should be, if you are in *any* doubt you must check with the nurse in charge.

Records and "hand-overs"

Information must flow throughout the care team. To ensure consistency and continuity of care, each member of that team needs to know what is going on. This means keeping effective records, and having regular "hand-overs" to exchange information between all those involved with the client's care. It will be up to the client, their key worker (or named nurse) and their care team to discuss and decide on what should be divulged to non-professional carers and relatives.

Records should be kept up to date. They should be securely stored to ensure confidentiality. Care assistants need to develop the skill and habit of recording their observations and what they have done in clear, concise and non-judgmental statements that can be understood by all, bearing in mind the client's right to see their own records. Each hospital or unit will have its own policy on how much writing on charts and records care assistants are expected to do.

Working as a team

It is important to remember you are part of a team. You probably work fewer than forty hours a week, but each client has one hundred and sixty eight hours of potential need a week, therefore it is clear that to address someone's needs properly the team must work together.

The care assistant's role within that team is a crucial one. You are generally the person who spends the most time with clients, and so you have access to the most information about individuals. Senior staff are generally responsible for clients' care, upkeep of records, liaising with relatives and other professionals, but they have many constraints upon their time, and must rely on care assistants for a good deal of "hands-on" care. Therefore it is imperative that care assistants share their experiences, thoughts and feelings with the senior members of staff.

Responsibilities are also worth considering. Senior staff are often accountable for all care activity within their area, so it is important that other staff recognise this and act accordingly. It is very important that instructions from senior staff are carried out accurately and promptly. If you are in any doubt about the reasons for the task you should question it, but unless you are satisfied that it is against the best interests of others or beyond your competency, you should complete the task. If you don't know, admit it and find out, but you should not just refuse to carry out an instruction.

Physical care

It is important to remember to treat each individual as a whole person, with both physical and psychological needs. This should be enshrined in the philosophy of any care environment, but can still be easily forgotten. Someone may be admitted with a psychiatric difficulty, but you must not forget to consider their physical needs and comforts as well. For instance a person feeling depressed may lose the will to eat or drink or attend to their basic hygiene. The care assistant must monitor their behaviour and encourage appropriate nutrition and hygiene, as well as addressing their depression.

General responsibilities

As well as your responsibility towards individual clients, you must always bear in mind your "corporate" obligations to others – not just other clients, but their relatives and carers, your colleagues and the public in general.

Policies and procedures: It is your responsibility to make sure you become familiar with local policies and procedures. Often these can be boring and laborious documents, but it is vital to remember they have not been created for nothing. Fire and security policies must be learned as soon as possible, as lives may depend on your knowledge and application of them. Others you may not need to know as fully, but they will provide useful information in often tricky situations.

Health and safety at work

As well as monitoring clients, it is also important that you monitor their environment. Part of your role is to ensure that the environment is maintained safely, and you must report anything you see as a risk to the nurse in charge. It may not be your job to mop up spilled tea, or fix a loose electrical plug, but it *is* your job to report such things to ensure they are done.

Health promotion: Anyone working in the care field has an important role in health promotion. "Modelling" appropriate behaviour is a powerful feature of this activity – that is displaying healthy and desirable behaviour and habits. After all is it reasonable to expect someone else to do something (stop smoking or lose weight for example) that you obviously do not?

Points to remember

1. Mental health care is concerned with addressing the needs of unique individuals.
2. Successful care is based on the care assistant's ability to understand and communicate effectively with their clients.
3. Good observation skills are crucial in mental health care.
4. Non-verbal communication skills are essential to good communication.
5. Communication with other staff, and teamwork, are fundamental to good care.
6. Awareness and care of the environment can be as important as individual care.

Suggested further reading

Manwatching by Desmond Morris, Triad Granada 1977.

The Naked Ape by Desmond Morris, Cape 1967.
Social Interaction by M.Argyle, Methuen 1978.
Stigma by I.Goffman, Penguin 1968.

NVQ Levels 2 & 3 Value Base Units
Ob Maintain confidentiality of information.
Oc Promote and support individual rights and choice within service delivery.
Od Acknowledge individuals' personal beliefs and identity.
Oe Support individuals through effective communication.

Levels 2 & 3 Core Units
U4 Contribute to the health, safety and security of individuals and their care environment.
U5 Obtain, transmit and store information relating to the delivery of a care service.

Level 2 Core Unit
W2 Contribute to the ongoing support of clients and others significant to them.

CHAPTER 18

Maternity care

Kim Turner

• Pregnancy and birth are stressful but normal life events – most mothers and babies are not ill • Health promotion and education • Monitoring • Emotional support • After the birth • The needs of the newborn baby: feeding, personal hygiene, sleeping, crying, love and attention

Pregnancy is a normal life event. Over 700,000 births occur each year in the United Kingdom. The purpose of the maternity service is to provide care for the woman and her family, from conception to 28 days after the birth.

In the normal course of events, this care is provided largely in the community setting. Most women give birth in a hospital setting and receive their first few days' postnatal care in hospital. However, for some women, care in hospital during pregnancy may be necessary.

But the vast majority of mothers and babies are not ill, and the role of health care workers in maternity wards has a different focus compared to many other areas of nursing. Care is focused towards promoting health and maintaining normality, while still acknowledging the crises women and their partners face throughout pregnancy, childbirth and the passage to parenthood.

Antenatal care

The majority of antenatal care is conducted in the community setting and the aim is to promote and maintain the health of the pregnant woman and her unborn child (fetus). Regular check-ups during pregnancy are designed to monitor the wellbeing of mother and fetus, prevent complications where possible, and to minimise any complications which do occur.

There are many physical, psychological, environmental and social factors which may complicate pregnancy and make admission to a maternity ward necessary. Women may be admitted simply for observation and investigation, and may sometimes require treatment. Pregnant women are as liable as any other group of people to develop illness or disease of any kind, but the fact that they are pregnant may alter the way in which the disease or illness shows itself, progresses and is treated. While there are standard factors in each case, the decisions taken and the eventual outcome will be different for every woman.

Key elements of care

Most women are self-caring and require few nursing interventions. Dependency levels vary according to the severity of their condition, but usually physical care is minimal. Care for these women centres around monitoring their condition, providing information and health education, and providing emotional and psychological support. All of these aspects of care enable women to make choices and take decisions about their care, making maternity care a partnership between the pregnant woman and the care staff.

Monitoring

The aim is to monitor progress, detect abnormal conditions and minimise complications. This is achieved through a variety of general and specific observations.

General observations include temperature, pulse and blood pressure recordings, urine testing, maternal weight assessment, dietary intake, fluid intake and output measurements and bowel habits. All of these fall within the role of the care assistant (see other chapters for more detail)

The specific observations include blood tests, abdominal examinations, fetal heart recordings, ultrasound examinations and vaginal examinations. The specific tests and examinations will fall outside the skills and role of the care assistant and will be performed by midwives and medical staff, but you may be required to assist in the preparation of equipment or to accompany the woman during the procedure.

All of these tests and recordings help to build up a picture of the general health and wellbeing of the mother and fetus, which will influence the management of the woman's care.

Information and health education

In order for women and their partners to be fully involved in their care and make decisions about that care, they need information. That information needs to be clear, unbiased, factual and accurate. It may range from what foods to eat during pregnancy, whether to have a particular screening test, which course of treatment to follow, what type of pain relief to use in labour, to termination of pregnancy.

Even in normal and uncomplicated pregnancies, women have to make complicated and difficult decisions. They are making decisions not only for themselves, but on behalf of their unborn child. Health care workers have a responsibility to enable women to make their own choices. The information may be passed to the woman on an individual basis or as part of formal antenatal classes. Pregnant women are very receptive and eager to learn how to care for themselves and their family. In this context, the care assistant has a role as a health educator. It is important that you understand the principles behind the information and advice given by the health professionals, and reinforce that information and advice when talking with pregnant women.

Emotional and psychological support

The importance of this aspect of maternity care must not be underestimated. Pregnant women have to cope with many physical, emotional and social changes in their lives. Pregnancy is a normal event but can be as stressful as moving house or getting divorced.

If the pregnancy is complicated, there is added stress and anxiety. A spell in the maternity ward may totally disrupt the woman's normal lifestyle. If a woman has experienced good health, then maternity care may be her first contact with a hospital environment. Her partner too is having to cope with changes and may be further stressed by concerns for his partner and child.

All of these factors influence how women and their partners behave and react with health professionals and may influence the care they receive. Social, religious and cultural differences are also important factors to be taken into consideration.

Communication and interpersonal skills – getting on with people – are vital aspects of the care assistant's role in maternity care, and as many areas of a woman's life may be investigated, confidentiality is a crucial issue (see also the section on gynaecology in chapter 13, chapter 2 on the responsibilities of the care assistant, and chapter 4 on communication).

A very large part of maternity care is psychological rather than physical. This means you are aiming to reduce fear and uncertainty, develop a working relationship with the woman and enhance relationships within her family, helping to prepare her for motherhood.

Care during labour

Throughout labour and birth, the woman will be cared for by midwives, supported by the obstetric and paediatric doctors. In the labour ward setting, the role of the care assistant centres around the support of the midwives rather than the care of the woman. You may be involved in preparing and maintaining the labour ward environment, preparing and maintaining charts and paperwork, answering the telephone, assisting with clinical procedures and preparing and serving food and drink. Your support is vitally important on the labour ward as it allows the midwives to devote their time and concentration to the woman herself and the progress of labour.

Postnatal care

Following birth, mothers spend a relatively short time in hospital before going home to the care of their general practitioner and community midwife.

Once again, the levels of dependency vary, but the majority of women and babies are not ill. If the birth has been straightforward, the woman is self-caring almost immediately and requires little physical care. Following a complicated birth, the woman requires additional care in the first few days but progresses to self-care very quickly. The woman may need your assistance with her personal hygiene (see Chapter 5) and in caring for her baby.

The aim of care in the postnatal period is to enable the mother to return to her pre-pregnant state of health, promote maternal and child health, establish infant feeding, develop the mother-infant relationship and prepare the mother and baby to join the rest of the family and the community.

Key Elements of Care

As in the antenatal period, care is based on three main elements:
• monitoring
• information and health education,
• emotional and psychological support

Mothers are encouraged to care fully for their infants from birth and therefore instruction in child care forms a major part of postnatal care.

Monitoring

Following birth, the woman's body begins to return to normal very quickly, and one aspect of care is to monitor that process. The mother's physical and psychological progress is monitored on a daily basis. The observations include temperature, blood pressure, pulse, dietary and fluid intake, bladder and bowel activity, examination of the breasts, abdomen and genitals, and assessment of blood loss. The physical checks are conducted by a midwife who uses the findings to pian care (see Care Plans, Chapter 1). An assessment is also made of the mother's psychological state

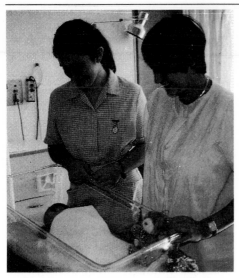

Babies, like their mothers, are individuals.

and how well she is adjusting to motherhood. Your role in this aspect of care is to undertake some of the monitoring, such as measurement of blood pressure, temperature, measuring fluid intake, recording that information and reporting findings and observations to the midwife in charge of the woman's care. This should also include observations of the woman's behaviour and her relationship with her family and baby. This will enable the midwife to make a full and accurate assessment of the woman's progress.

Information and health education
The woman's progress is enhanced by promoting health and minimising complications. This may be achieved through encouraging a healthy lifestyle; personal hygiene, adequate diet, achieving a balance between rest and exercise, use of relaxation techniques, and health education surrounding women's health issues such as breast screening and family planning.

The role of parents also brings with it the responsibility of making decisions on behalf of the infant. New parents are faced with many choices and decisions to make. Their need for information is overwhelming, ranging from whether to use disposable or terry nappies, to whether or not to accept recommended drugs and immunisations for the infant.

The focus of care is towards enabling the parents to make their own decisions. You can help by reinforcing the information and advice given by the midwives and and medical staff and by talking with women, allowing them to express their anxieties and consider their options. If the woman or her partner needs more information or asks questions that you cannot answer, you must refer to the midwife. It is important that you do not attempt to give a level of care, or advice, beyond the scope of your training and competence (see Ch. 1).

Emotional and psychological support
Following childbirth, 1 in 10 women will experience depression to a greater or lesser degree. Support and empathy from health professionals and care assistants can help women ease into their new role as mothers, preventing and reducing the devastating effects of severe postnatal depression. While partners do not officially suffer from postnatal depression, their need for support and empathy can be just as great.

Your role here may be as simple as merely lending a listening ear, while also observing the woman's behaviour and attitude. While you need to maintain the woman's privacy and confidentiality, you must also report your observations and any information which may influence the woman's care, to the midwife.

Child care
Many women and their partners have little practical experience of caring for babies and young children. Practical instruction and health promotion issues form the basis of this aspect of maternity

care. This may range from advice on infant feeding, environmental issues and prevention of cot death, to the recognition of normal development patterns. The focus again is to enable the parents to assume full responsibility for the care of their infant. Your role ranges from helping the mother with the practical aspects of child care to providing information and discussing options with her.

The needs of the newborn

The needs of the newborn are simple; warmth, food, personal hygiene, sleep, love and attention. Providing for all the infant's needs promotes growth and development. Babies, like their mothers, are individuals and while their needs and progress follow similar patterns, caring for them is far from routine. You will be involved in their actual care alongside the midwives and other members of the multidisciplinary team, but the baby belongs to the parents and the focus of care is to enable parenting skills and parental responsibility to develop.

Feeding

Most women have decided early on in pregnancy how to feed their baby. Over 70 per cent of women choose to breast feed. Breast feeding is a natural and normal process but women need instruction, guidance, support and encouragement in order to establish a good milk supply and to continue feeding. This includes advice on nursing bras, care of the breasts, how to prevent problems, how to deal with problems, how and when to feed and how to express and store milk.

You can support breastfeeding mothers by reinforcing the advice and information given by the midwife and by offering practical assistance, for example helping her to get comfortable before and during a feed.

Women who choose to bottle feed also need instruction, guidance and support. This includes advice on the range of milks available, the equipment needed, sterilisation techniques, and how and when to feed.

Whether women choose to breast or bottle feed, feeding the baby on demand is encouraged, letting the baby lead the feeding and allowing him/her to settle into a personal routine.

Personal hygiene

Babies need to be cleansed and bathed in order to prevent infection. Bathing, "top and tail" (face and bottom washing) and napkin changing techniques are all part of the parents' education. They are also an important factor in stimulating the infant's development as they provide a time when baby and parent can communicate and develop their relationship.

Sleeping

Babies' sleep patterns vary a great deal and their personal sleep pattern develops over a period of time. Current research into cot death recommends that babies are placed on their back when laid down to sleep. This position is known to reduce the incidence of cot death.

Crying

This is the baby's main method of communication and as it can take parents some time to learn their baby's language, crying is a major source of distress for new parents. Babies rarely cry for no reason and there are many different types of cry. It takes time for parents to distinguish what their baby's cries mean and they will need guidance and support in learning to understand their infant.

Love and attention

Babies need physical, psychological and emotional stimulation as an aid to normal development. Parents need guidance and encouragement in order to fully develop their relationship with the infant. Through learning about their baby as an individual, they help to develop his or her personality and achieve the develop-mental milestones such as smiling, reaching, holding, walking and talking.

Part of the team

In maternity wards, the role of the care assistant as a support worker is just that, supportive, but in a very active manner. By providing nursing care, undertaking clerical and domestic tasks, communicating with clients and staff, offering guidance and education to clients, you will be supporting the whole structure of the maternity service – supporting women, supporting their families and supporting the midwives and medical staff. This supportive but active role will help provide a quality service designed to meet the needs of its customers.

Points to remember

1. Pregnancy is a normal life event.
2. There are many physical, psychological, social, environmental, cultural and religious factors which may influence a woman's experience of pregnancy, childbirth and motherhood.
3. Women have a right to choose, for themselves and on behalf of their babies.
4. Hospital-based care is usually a short episode in the cycle of pregnancy, birth and parenthood.
5. Maternity care extends beyond the confines of the maternity wards, involving the woman's family and the community.
6. Mothers and babies are individuals. They are not only our customers but our future society; they expect and deserve a good service.

NVQ Levels 2 & 3 Value Base Units

Ob Maintain confidentiality of information.
Oc Promote and support individual rights and choice within service delivery.
Od Acknowledge individuals' personal beliefs and identity.
Oe Support individuals through effective communication.

Levels 2 & 3 Core Units

U4 Contribute to the health, safety and security of individuals and their care environment.
U5 Obtain, transmit and store information relating to the delivery of a care service.

Level 2 Core Unit

W2 Contribute to the ongoing support of clients and other significant to them. environment.
W3 Support clients in transition due to their care requirements.

Level 2 Postnatal Care Endorsement

Z16 - Care for a baby in the first 10 days of life when the mother is unable.
W6 - Reinforce professional advice through supporting and encouraging the mother in active parenting in first 10 days of baby's life.

CHAPTER 19

Caring for children in hospital

Esther Parker

• The special skills you need • A different kind of ward environment • Family-centred care • Admission – planned and emergency • The importance of play, and education • Special aspects of care • Talking and listening to children • The child facing death

Caring for children in hospital takes a special kind of person and requires a variety of very specialist skills. These include a range of communication and interpersonal skills, observation skills and patience.

Children become ill very quickly, and their condition can get worse extremely rapidly. So it is vitally important that you pass on as soon as possible any changes you observe in a child's condition, to the nurse coordinating their care. On the other hand children also tend to recover at the same speed, and will be up and about more quickly than you would expect of an adult.

Bright and noisy

Children's wards are usually brightly coloured units, with pictures, murals and posters decorating the walls and windows. A large range of toys and books is visible, and there is a constant background of music or videos. The patients spend a minimum amount of time in bed, and when they are up they normally wear their own clothes.

Often a parent, usually Mum, is "resident", staying with their child. Some wards have special facilities but for many parents this involves sleeping in a folding bed alongside the child's bed or cot. Open visiting – visits at any time of day from parents, brothers, sisters, and, especially for the adolescent, friends – is encouraged.

Many of these changes came about after health professionals recognised the importance of **family centred care.** This means seeing the child as part of a family unit, and that the needs of the family will influence the needs of the child. It is also considered essential to involve the child's family, as well as the child, in the planning and giving of care. This is often referred to as a "partnership of care" or **parental participation**.

It is important to remember that the parent's capacity to be involved in care giving should be negotiated, never assumed. It must also be reviewed regularly as the parent's ability to contribute may increase or decrease as a result of changes, particularly in the child's condition, home or work pressures.

Planned admission

The child either has a planned admission to hospital or is admitted as a result of an emergency.

For a planned, or "elective" admission the parents are aware of the coming admission and will usually have taken time to prepare the child. The family may even have taken part in a pre-admission programme that many children's wards run, involving a visit to the ward, watching a video, taking part in play-orientated activity and having an opportunity to ask questions. While the child and their parents may still be apprehensive and unsure, they should be aware of what is likely to happen during their stay.

These children are usually well, so with open visiting and shorter admissions, staff can find it difficult to keep track of who is the patient and who is just visiting! Particular care needs to be taken to identify who is allowed to eat and who is being starved in preparation for theatre or an investigation. This is important, as some children and relatives think that "not eating and drinking" doesn't mean they can't have crisps and sweets.

Emergency admission

The needs of the child who is admitted as an emergency are two-fold. Firstly, the child's condition must be assessed and the appropriate nursing care given, keeping the child safe. The measuring and recording of vital signs, such as temperature, pulse, breathing rate and blood pressure, is an important part of this. Information can also be gathered through observing skin colour, posture, movement, how they relate and react to adults and their parents. Do report and document any changes or anything unusual. Parents are a vital source of information regarding changes in condition and differences from the child's normal pattern of behaviour. Do ask and involve them.

The second need is to relieve anxiety in both parent and child, by supporting them, giving reassurance and gradually familiarising them with the ward surroundings and facilities.

Play

Play is said to be the child's work, and is an important part of the child's daily activity. For young children it is a way of exploring and making sense of the world around them. It is also a part of the child's developmental process, allowing the development of various motor skills, such as running, skipping and jumping, as well as the fine skills which include holding and using a pencil or crayon, doing up a button and manipulating small objects.

If a child has to be immobile for any length of time, this developmental process needs to be continued by making sure that a range of play materials is brought to the child, to stimulate and challenge their ability.

Everyday activities should not be overlooked. Much fun, as well as skill, can be gained while rolling out pastry for jam tarts or peeling carrots and potatoes. Finding a story book that also involves the same activity can bring a touch of normality to the child's life.

Play can help to prepare a child for theatre or other procedures using play material, anatomical dolls or art work. Not only can the child be given an explanation of what is going to happen, but through play the child is often able to express worries that they would not otherwise be able to put into words.

As the child gets older play takes other roles. It continues to develop skills and allow a safety net for expressing feelings and concerns. The socialisation that occurs through play becomes very important, initially confined to a close group of family and friends, but then widening, drawing in others.

Play can also be used in a number of ways as a therapeutic tool, particularly to work through upsetting or traumatic experiences and to encourage a child to participate in physically beneficial activities. Riding a tricycle or pedal car can be more fun than doing exercises to develop leg muscles or loosen a stiffened joint. Blowing a pea along with a straw or blowing up balloons is an effective way of getting a child to do deep breathing. Learning through play can be a way of coming to terms with the requirements and unit counting involved in a diabetic diet, in the same way that spelling and familiarity with numbers can be improved by games such as Scrabble and others involving score keeping.

As the child becomes older, play becomes more of a time filler and may develop into a hobby. Often the older child sees play as a more structured activity, involving formal games that have defined rules, like team sports.

Changes in a child's normal type of play may clearly indicate how the child feels and the stage of their recovery. Children often need help in adjusting to a different form of play. A child who is used to active, unstructured play involving large areas will find playing in bed restrictive. Likewise a child who is used to solo, quiet play may find the ward environment very daunting.

During play, the child's safety must be protected. Physical safety means recognising potential hazards and making sure toys are appropriate for the age group of the child. There should be no sharp ends or loose pieces for young children and babies who are likely to put them into their mouths. Children must also be protected emotionally, and not be forced into play that would upset them.

Schooling

The child's education is continued even during hospital admission. Normally, lessons are given to all except very ill children. They go to a school room or area, even when confined to bed, or work is brought to their bedside. Older children and those in hospital for extended periods are encouraged to maintain links with their own school, continuing the same work as their class so that they do not fall behind with their studies. This is very important for the child who has regular or frequent admissions.

Giving care

Aspects of physical care are covered in other chapters, but there are important points to remember in caring for children:

• Always explain to the child what you are going to do before you do it, just as you would with an adult, but make sure your explanation is in language appropriate for their age and level of understanding.

• Help is often required in feeding, or cutting food up so that a child can eat independently. Food should always be presented in small but attractive portions, on a small plate. Large portions will just make a child reluctant to eat. Small cups, partially filled, are safer than a large cup or glass. Do make sure that neither food nor drink is too hot. Accurate recording, especially of fluids taken, may be important.

• When lifting and moving a child do take as much care as you would if moving a larger person or weight (see Chapter 7). Children rarely help, so you lift a dead weight that may wriggle.

Talking to children

Nurses and care assistants frequently have to teach the child and their family to understand a condition they may have to live with for most or all of their life. There are two key principles: ALWAYS talk to a child in language appropriate to their age and understanding, and NEVER lie to them. It takes a long time to regain the trust of a child who has discovered they have not been told the truth. In some cases the relationship never recovers.

Language development
As a child gets older their understanding and language skills also develop. By toddler age, the child can usually say a number of words but can understand or recognise many more. Words are often repeated and simple commands obeyed, but there is no understanding of right and wrong.

The "why" stage is reached at about three years old. But although questions are asked, the answers are frequently ignored as the child's attention quickly wanders. Simple explanations need to be given in response. Time has little relevance, so "hold on" or "just a minute" is not understood.

By school age the range of vocabulary has greatly increased. The child begins to recognise time span, normally in relation to meals and sleep. They still remain very egocentric – **I** or **me** is what is important. But they are very

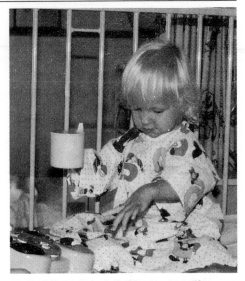

By toddler age, a child can usually say a number of words but understand many more.

imaginative and will often involve their teddy or another object to explain how they feel. This involvement can also be used when giving an explanation or teaching the child. Pictures can also be useful.

Around the age of seven, the child is beginning to develop a more realistic view of the world. While they now realise that there can be an alternative view, things are seen very much as either right or wrong. Disease or illness is something that just happens and they can be very matter of fact about a situation that an adult may find quite distressing. Explanations needed to be related to everyday things as children at this stage cannot yet form mental images. Lungs, for example, can be portrayed as an upside down tree, with trunk and branches as the "breathing tubes".

In the early teenage years abstract thought and the ability to formalise, rationalise and test out opinion develop, but these children still have very definite ideas and see things as being either black or white with little grey area between.

Teaching

Teaching a child is a skill that takes a lot of practice. It is important to break the topic down into a logical order and present any facts in a simple but informative manner. Even a teenager will find it easier to take information in when it is linked to current hobby or interest. After any explanation, do not ask a child, "Do you understand?", as the answer will usually be yes. Instead ask them to explain it to you. That way you can check just what information has been taken in and that it is correct. (See also Chapter 3, Talking and Listening).

The child facing death

The same ability to understand is relevant when talking to the child facing death, either their own or that of a close relative. Younger children can be so matter of fact, their frankness can be very disconcerting. Death is just an inevitable part of life to them and anyone they see as "grown up" is old to them. It can also be seen as a solution to the discomfort and pain that they are experiencing.

The older child needs sensitive handling, with the opportunity to talk through feelings and frustrations. Realisation that ambitions and relationships will never be achieved is also an important area to be explored. However, this can never be rushed and the child must decide when and where is the right time to discuss these issues.

Always make time if the child wants to talk. Once they have made the decision or the approach it is usually impossible to "save it until later". This is certainly true for the young child, but is equally important to remember when working with the older child.

Points to remember

1. Do involve the child and family in all stages of care.
2. Always tell the child what you are going to do, in language appropriate to their age.
3. A child's condition can change rapidly. Always report and record changes in condition immediately.
4. Play is an important activity for a child.
5. Children often find it difficult to talk about their fears and worries. It is very important to allow them time to talk when they need it.

NVQ Levels 2 & 3 Value Base Units
Oc Promote and support individual rights and choice within service delivery.
Oe Support individuals through effective communication.

Levels 2 & 3 Core Units
U4 Contribute to the health, safety and security of individuals and their care environment.
U5 Obtain, transmit and store information relating to the delivery of a care service.

Level 2 Core Unit
W2 Contribute to the ongoing support of clients and others significant to them. environment.
W3 Support clients in transition due to their care requirements.
Z10 Enable clients to eat and drink.

Level 2 Special Care Needs Endorsement
Z13. Enable clients to participate in recreation and leisure activities.

NVQ Level 3 Acute Care (Children)
X19 Prepare and undertake agreed ongoing clinical activities with clients in acute care settings.
Z8 Support clients when they are distressed.

CHAPTER 20

Care for people with learning disabilities

Margaret Whoriskey and Carol Welch

• Community care and the forgotten hospitals • The challenge for care staff • Special needs, challenging behaviour, elderly people, dementia • Planning care for individuals • Working within the multi-disciplinary team • Your role and relationships • Quality assurance • Life beyond the hospital

Over recent years in the UK, the aim agreed by all agencies involved in long term care of people with learning disabilities has been that services should be based on the principle of "normalisation". This means simply that they should live and be cared for in small residential homes in a district where their families and friends live, rather than in the large hospitals, mostly built in the last century, set apart in their own grounds away from everyday community life. The assumption is that care in small homes within the community will lead to a better and more normal lifestyle for people with learning disabilities.

So for years now the aim has been to discharge residents to the "community" and run down the large institutions. In some areas this has been achieved, but the task of closing hospitals has not been as easy as was originally thought.

The forgotten hospitals?

Most people agree that life in a large institution is far from ideal. The reality, however, is that for a number of people with learning disabilities, hospital will remain their home for the foreseeable future. There are also cases (although few) of new admissions to hospitals, where community services have not been able to meet their needs.

But while residents and staff remain there, resources have trickled out from hospitals over the years, leaving them feeling forgotten and "left behind".

The challenge

Care assistants need to accept the challenge of an uncertain future during this long-running transition from hospital to community living, developing a positive view and a sense of value in their role.

Many years ago our hospitals accommodated large numbers of residents at all levels of ability, but with the move towards community care, most if not all the people with a very mild learning disability have left, often to live independently or with minimal support.

Residents currently in a hospital setting tend to be more severely disabled, often with additional physical problems and/or difficult behaviour. The range of needs is wide and people with learning disabilities do not form a uniform group.

Many hospitals have tried to identify residents according to their predominant need. For example:

Special needs

This is a term used to describe people with a severe or profound disability who often have complicated medical conditions, such as epilepsy. They may be deaf and/or blind and have very little communication. Because of the excellent medical care now available, a number of people who previously would not have survived are living, often well into adulthood and old age.

Challenging behaviour

This is now a well used and familiar phrase to describe people whose behaviour is very difficult for us to tolerate or manage.

It is not always possible to say what causes the behaviour; it may be due to a combination of factors such as the extent of the brain damage, lack of appropriate communication and other skills, and environmental factors.

Because of the number of staff working in a hospital setting it is difficult for all staff to respond to residents in the same way. At times this can mean that "problem" behaviour is being reacted to differently and there is not a consistent way of dealing with it.

There are also a few residents who, in addition to their learning disability, have a mental illness. Sometimes this gives rise to behaviour that is difficult to manage.

Elderly people

There is a rapidly increasing group of elderly people within the general population and this is also the case in the area of learning disability. Years ago it was unusual to see people with learning disabilities in their 70s and 80s, but it is now more commonplace and we need to be able to respond to the needs of this group.

Dementia

Some elderly people will develop a dementia (see chapter 16), causing severe memory problems and confused behaviour. Research has shown also that a number of people with Down's Syndrome can develop dementia at a much younger age than is usual, in their 30s and 40s. The needs of this group will again be quite different and place different demands on the care assistant.

Individuals

Many residents in hospital do not fall neatly into a specific category of need. They will in fact have a range of disabilities and skills which require an individual approach to their care. Two commonly-used ways of ensuring that the resident is considered first and foremost as an individual, are *Nursing Care Plans* (explained in Chapter 5), and *Individual Programme Planning (IPP)*, which has a more multidisciplinary focus.

Individual Programme Plans

Individual Programme Plans, or IPPs as they are more commonly known, were developed to ensure a co-ordinated multidisciplinary individual plan for people with learning disabilities. The system is probably more often used in community settings but a number of hospitals are implementing IPPs.

An Individual Programme Plan involves the individual resident as fully as possible along with their relatives, care staff and other professionals such as speech therapist, occupational therapist, consultant psychiatrist and so on. An individual's strengths (that is, what skills, interests, relationships, likes, etc they have) and their needs are assessed by care staff and others and a plan is then developed on the basis of this. The nursing care plan assessment will contribute to this process.

A number of goals – both short term (over the next few months) and long term (over the next year or more) – are set and reviewed on a regular basis. A key worker or named nurse is identified for each individual resident, and in many cases this is a care assistant. The key worker has a "special" relationship with the individual, and can be responsible for co-ordinating that person's IPP.

An IPP should cover all aspects of a person's life, from medical needs to financial issues, to how an individual can be helped to develop social relationships, and skills they require to learn.

The key worker must know the individual well and meet them often. A useful book for further information on this system of working is *Individual Programme Planning*[1].

The multidisciplinary team

Earlier chapters of this book have outlined the role of the care assistant within the hospital setting and in relation to other disciplines, and this is largely relevant to the care assistant working in a hospital for people with learning disabilities. However, because of the range of needs there are often a confusing number of other staff involved. The care assistant, who may be the identified key worker, can feel swamped by this, particularly if it hasn't been made clear who is doing what.

The process of Individual Programme Planning described above helps to avoid confusion and duplication and should help in identifying the multi-disciplinary team. Membership of the team will include a number of health professionals such as consultant psychiatrist, nursing staff, physiotherapist, clinical psychologist, occupational therapist, speech therapist, dietitian and in some hospitals, people such as art, drama or music therapists.

In addition, there will be staff who

NAME: John SMITH	Individual Programme Plan
Strengths Has good communication skills Has regular contact with his family Can travel on public transport with supervision Carries out personal hygiene with prompting Enjoys country and western music	*Needs* To phone his family once a week To learn to travel on public transport independently To initiate shaving every morning
Goal statement - John will travel independently on the bus from the hospital to the country and western club once a week.	

Example of a strengths and needs list and goal statement from an Individual Programme Plan.

provide day care and also staff from other agencies such as teachers and social workers who will have some involvement with the individual resident. No wonder we feel swamped!

As a care assistant you may feel anxious about contributing to discussion when there are so many other people involved. However, it is often the care assistant who knows the individual resident best – their likes, dislikes, how they react to changes – and your view can be most valuable. It is care assistants who have the one to one close contact with residents, therefore it is you who can enhance and enrich the lives of the people in your care by your attitude and your actions.

Your role and relationships

The role of the care assistant in a hospital for people with learning disabilities is varied and demanding. The range of needs of this client group requires a flexible and enthusiastic approach, and the caring role can vary from one day to the next.

Because the hospital is also their home for most residents, it is important to realise that staff come to mean a lot to the residents. In the absence of involved relatives, residents have little opportunity to develop meaningful relationships and can become very attached to care staff. This can often be reciprocal although it is important to be aware of becoming over involved. Good support and guidelines from other nursing staff will usually avoid any problems.

Because care staff have to perform a number of roles the skills required are numerous. Staff training, along with good supervision, should assist in carrying out the duties of the job well and with a positive attitude.

There are many roles a care assistant may fulfil in the hospital setting for people with learning disabilities, such as:

Physical care

As increasing numbers of residents remaining in hospital require physical care, a considerable amount of time will be spent on tasks common to all areas of care, such as:
- lifting and handing
- personal care and hygiene
- feeding procedures
- providing a comfortable and safe environment
- communicating with residents and helping them to communicate their needs and feelings
- implementing, under supervision, the plan for care.

Key Workers

A number of hospitals and community based services operate a Key Worker system which has been described briefly in the section on Individual Programme Planning. Usually the care assistant will be the Key Worker for a number of individuals in the ward. This means they will be the person who is responsible for the overall well being of the resident(s). This role includes:
- getting to know the individual resident and being able to identify their strengths, needs and wishes
- liaising with other staff and relatives
- contributing to the assessment process
- supporting the resident and representing their wishes if possible. Often people with learning disabilities lack confidence and it is the care worker's place to speak on their behalf or help them to speak up for themselves.

Teaching

Many staff do not consider themselves teachers or instructors, but very often the job involves encouraging residents to learn new skills and follow teaching programmes developed for the resident.

The range of skills the care assistant can be involved in teaching will be many, but can include:

• toilet training
• personal care and hygiene
• feeding
• road crossing
• use of shops, public transport, etc.

Obviously the type of skills being taught will vary according to the level of ability of the resident. In addition to "formal" teaching programmes that may be carried out at certain times, there are many opportunities throughout the day to provide more informal teaching by:
• you being a role model – setting a good example in carrying out certain activities;
• prompting and encouraging the resident to be as independent as possible. Even allowing the resident to make simple choices about food, activities, and so on will assist in the learning process.

These roles will merge a lot of the time and staff are not necessarily conscious of what particular hat they are wearing when involved in a specific task. However it is important to be aware of the range of roles you are required to fulfil as you work.

Quality assurance

Many hospitals will now have a range of policies and quality standards to ensure a better quality service for residents and staff. Many of these are similar to those in other hospital settings – health and safety, smoking, etc. But because of the nature of the work in learning disabilities, other policies have emerged, such as:

• residents rights
• policies on relationships and sexuality
• Individual Programme Planning (discussed earlier)

This has come about because of the recognition that although clients in our services are vulnerable and need protection, they have the same rights as the rest of us.

Quality standards are now a feature of the National Health Service and staff are encouraged to develop their own standards as relevant to their ward or setting. By setting standards we ensure consistency in care for our residents.

All staff involved in care can assure the quality of the service they provide by simply reading the standards for their particular ward or department and working to achieve them. Standards can be applied to all areas of care and all levels and grades of staff can participate in producing standards.

There are three stages in writing a standard.

1. What you need - STRUCTURE
2. How you do it - PROCESS
3. What you want
      to achieve - OUTCOME
An example is shown opposite.

It is important that standards are monitored and reviewed regularly.

Staff training

By now you may feel that the job involves a great deal of knowledge and expertise, although many people have been doing it for years and doing it very well. Most hospitals have a system of training, both for new staff and to update everyone on new procedures.

Induction Training
When you take up a post as care assistant, many hospitals will ensure that you are given a period of training before you work on the ward. Induction Training

Right: An example of a Quality Standard that directly affects the care of residents.

FIFE HEALTH BOARD

STANDARD REF. NO	Any ward	01/111	ACHIEVE STANDARD BY	1st May 1994
TOPIC	Individualised care		REVIEW STANDARD BY	1st Oct 1994
SUB TOPIC	Well fitting footwear		SIGNATURE OF DNS	
CARE GROUP	All residents		SIGNATURE OF SENIOR NURSE	
SOURCE OF INFORMATION	C/N Jones/Ms Smith CMN		DATE	1st Jan 1994

STANDARD STATEMENT: Each resident has well-fitting shoes, which are comfortable to wear and suited to their needs

STRUCTURE

Training: All staff should -
Be educated on the importance of well-fitting shoes and the importance of residents wearing them at the appropriate times.

Each resident to have feet measured by an experienced shoe fitter.

Nurse has knowledge of how to contact chiropodist.

Guidelines: Information on foot development and the importance of wearing correct footwear to be available on the ward (brochures, leaflets etc).

All staff to be made aware of damage that can be caused if incorrect footwear is applied.

Availability of staff: Staff who are experienced in dealing with special footwear are available to demonstrate to all staff the correct method of applying the footwear and the importance of this.

PROCESS

1. The nurse with the help of the physiotherapist to assess residents who would benefit from specially adapted shoes.

2. All special needs regarding footwear and progress to be recorded in residents' profiles. To be assessed and re-assessed at regular intervals.

3. The nurse contacts the physiotherapy department for help when required.

4. All nursing staff to ensure that residents have the correct footwear.

OUTCOME

1. Each resident will have footwear which is: well-fitting, comfortable to wear and suited to their individual needs.

2. All nurses will have had sufficient instruction on the importance of each resident having the correct footwear.

3. Foot care will be of a much higher standard and quality.

4. Footwear will be clearly marked so there is no mistaking whose footwear is whose.

programmes tend to vary from hospital to hospital, although all will have a basic core of information which you must learn before you are allowed to work on a ward. Topics covered may include:

- lifting and handling techniques
- bed making
- bathing
- general nursing care
- how to handle aggression
- feeding disabled residents
- epilepsy

In-service Training

Most hospitals will have a programme of regular staff training to update staff on issues, new procedures and policies.

Life beyond the hospital

While this chapter has looked at the role of the care assistant within the hospital setting, the skills and experience will be relevant to community based services, and staff should not feel anxious about transferring from one setting to the other. The new services will benefit from the knowledge and background of care staff who come from a hospital setting, often with years of valuable experience and expertise.

Points to remember

1. Many people will continue to live in a hospital setting until more appropriate services are developed in the community.
2. The needs of residents will vary from total dependency on others for day-to-day care, to more able residents who may also have a mental illness and/or display challenging behaviour.
3. The care assistant is a member of the multi-disciplinary team and your opinion can make a valuable contribution to the care of the person.
4. The role of the care assistant requires a range of skills, from caring to teaching and representing residents' views and wishes.
5. Staff training is a key component to providing a good quality service.
6. There is life beyond the hospital and many care staff should consider using their skills in the new services being developed in the community.

NVQ Value Base Units

Oc Promote and support individual rights and choice within service delivery.
Od Acknowledge individuals' personal beliefs and identities.

Levels 2 & 3 Core Units

U5 Obtain, transmit and store information relating to the delivery of a care service.

Level 2 Special Care Needs Endorsement

X1 Contribute to the support of clients during development programmes and activities.
W8 Enable clients to maintain contacts in potentially isolating situations.

Further reading

1. *Individual Programme Planning*, by Judith Jenkins et al, BILD Publications 1988. British Institute of Learning Disabilities, Wolverhampton Rd, Kidderminster, Worcs DY10 3PP. Tel: 0562 850251.

A Practical Guide to Working With People with Learning Disabilities - A Handbook for Care Assistants and Support Workers, edited by Hilary Brown and Sue Benson, Hawker Publications, 13 Park House, 140 Battersea Park Road, London SW11 4NB. Tel: 071 720 2108.

CHAPTER 21

Stress in your life and your work

Michael Wafer

• What is stress and how does it affect us? • Stress in hospital work • Causes of stress • How to recognise and cope with stress in your life and stressful situations at work • The patient's point of view • Special problems for women

Stress in recent years has become a "buzz" word, a topic frequently discussed in our daily newspapers and television programmes. There seems to be a general view in our society that life today is more stressful than it was many years ago. But what is stress?

We all know what it is when we experience it, but may have difficulty defining it. The word is derived from "distress", and when we use it in a day-to-day sense, we may think of being under pressure, under strain, and lacking energy.

In a medical sense the term means the release of chemicals within the body, providing it with extra energy for either "fight or flight". In primitive times, if a person felt threatened in his surroundings the body would respond by providing extra energy to allow them either to run away or to fight.

In our day-to-day life we also have threatening experiences. An example might be going to the dentist: our primitive response to the threat is to run away, and our body provides us with the chemicals to enable us to do this. Most of us, however, remain sitting in the chair.

Even though the body does not use those chemicals which allow us to escape, they are still released and have an effect on the body. An example of an illness caused by the release of these chemicals is stomach ulcers. Indeed it is recognised that many modern diseases are caused in part by stress.

Stress can also be pleasurable and useful to a person. We might feel stressed when watching a horror movie, or riding on a roller coaster, or watching our favourite team in the Wembley final. Or at work, you might have to cope with several events at the same time, such as the admission of several patients in a short period of time. When feeling stressed we sometimes give our best performance as we get a "burst of adrenalin". This type of beneficial stress is sometimes called *eustress*.

Stress in hospitals

It is generally accepted that working in hospitals can be stressful. It is not difficult to see why. Some causes of stress are to do with the nature of the work, such as the close contact with people who are suffering pain, or may be depressed, or dying. Other examples may be working shifts, low pay, or poor working conditions. In addition to all this there have been tremendous changes in the health service which have caused feelings of uncertainty, and fear of job loss, which have given rise to further stress.

These feelings of stress have very important consequences. They may make people less effective in their work, and so the care they give others may suffer. Stress at work may also affect people's personal lives and close relationships. It is therefore in everyone's interest that stress is understood, and that we try to find ways to limit its harmful effects.

What causes stress?

Researchers have tried to identify **events in life** which are particularly stressful. These include, in order of severity:

• Death of partner
• Divorce or separation
• Death of close family member
• Marriage
• Loss of job
• Gain of new family member
• Financial problems
• Change in housing
• Change of job

If you have experienced one or more of the above within the last twelve months it is likely that you have felt under some degree of stress.

Examples of **work situations** which may make you feel stressed are:

• Dealing with seriously ill patients
• Not feeling valued as a member of the team

• Being asked to do tasks for which you have not been adequately trained
• Difficult relationships with senior members of staff
• Sexual harassment
• Witnessing bad practice

In addition to the above there are many other factors in the hospital workplace which can make us feel stressed. These include difficult staff relations, medical emergencies, and too much noise.

A particular problem for the care assistant is that because of your position in the organisation you may feel relatively powerless, that you have no control over the things which are putting you under strain. The truth is, of course, that you do have control over what happens to you at work, and you can influence the people around you and the environment. Some of the ways you can do this will be discussed later.

Recognising stress

If you are suffering from stress, your body will tell you! Some of the physical symptoms include feeling sick, sweating, going to the toilet more often, irregular periods, constipation, dry mouth, inability to sleep, indigestion, eating more or eating less, headaches, and palpitations.

In addition to physical symptoms you may have alteration in mood. You may cry more easily, feel down and depressed, feel anxious, feel inadequate, feel negative, or feel hysterical.

You may not be able to think clearly. You may lack concentration, you may not be able to make decisions, you may feel that your life is totally out of control.

Stress may also be evident from a change of behaviour. This might include absenteeism, arriving late for work, increased smoking and drinking, being withdrawn and quiet, inappropriate laughter, being aggressive, or being clumsy. Sometimes it will be other people who recognise that you are under stress, before you do.

Coping with stress

In trying to cope with stress there are three broad approaches. The first of these is to try and live your life in such a way that your body is not exposed to unpleasant and unnecessary stress. The second is that if you are suffering from stress you try to identify the cause, and either eliminate or reduce it. Finally you can try and deal with the feelings produced by stress.

Lifestyle

In order to reduce stress you should try and lead a healthy lifestyle. This includes paying attention to your diet – not only should this be "balanced" (including a wide variety of good food) but you should not miss meals. This can be particularly difficult for people working in hospitals because of the irregular hours and shift work. Try to reduce your intake of tea and coffee (or drink decaffeinated drinks) as caffeine is a stimulant and may contribute to your feeling stressed.

It is important that you get enough sleep. Allow for adequate rest times: if you have any influence on work rotas try to avoid working for long periods without days off, similarly try to take holidays at equally spaced intervals.

Exercise is very important. Not only will it make you fitter, it will help you work off stressful feelings and also help you sleep better.

In addition to a healthy lifestyle it is important to find ways to relax, and to make time in the day to carry out that

relaxation. Methods of relaxing are very personal but might include listening to music, or going for a walk.

Talk to someone

A very important way of relieving and preventing stress is to talk to people. Find a suitable time to confide in someone you trust about the parts of your life which are making you feel stressed. Sometimes friends and partners may provide all the support you need, but they may find it difficult to understand work-related problems if they have never worked in a hospital. Often work colleagues can be very supportive.

Some hospitals provide either counselling within the occupational health service or alternatively independent counsellors. In addition you may find some of the voluntary organisations helpful, for example MIND (the National Association for Mental Health), Relate (Marriage Guidance), and the Samaritans, whose local numbers should be found in the Yellow Pages telephone directory.

Find the cause

If you are feeling stressed you should try to identify the cause. You cannot always remove the cause of stress, of course, but in some instances you can. You may be feeling stressed because of high noise levels for example, which you may be able to reduce.

A common cause of stress is difficulty with colleagues; if this is the case it is important that you discuss it with the person concerned. In the short term it may feel very uncomfortable, but it is likely to have long term benefits.

Smoking and drinking

Unfortunately many of us deal with the problems of stress by dealing with the symptoms. This may include increasing our alcohol intake, or smoking more. It may have the effect of us feeling better for a brief period, but once the drink has gone the problem will still be there (and may be made worse by a hangover).

Stress in the workplace

Perhaps the single most important factor in reducing stress in the workplace is the development of good relationships between workers. This is very easy to write down, but I suspect many of us would agree it can be difficult to achieve.

An important element of good working relationships is **trust**. The following will destroy trust:

• talking critically behind people's backs
• breaking confidences
• breaking agreements
• trying to manipulate people for your own ends
• being inconsistent
• reporting to a senior person without discussion with the person concerned first.

Trust can be developed in many ways, including:

• being honest and saying what you think without being aggressive or negatively critical
• Openly expressing your support for people you work with
• sharing information
• listening to advice given
• helping everybody feel valued for their contribution to the team.

It is important that you try to do something about the things that you find stressful. A particularly difficult area is if you witness **bad practice**. An example might be the maltreatment of a patient (including verbal abuse). It is important that you discuss this with the staff member concerned, and report it to the person immediately senior to you. Physical abuse *must* be reported to the person in charge immediately. If you fail to do this not only will you feel stressed, but you will be collaborating by failing to report the incident and allowing someone to continue to carry out bad practice.

If you cannot personally control or change stressful factors in the workplace it is important that you report them to someone who can. In most hospital wards this could be the ward sister or charge nurse.

Stress and patients

Studies have shown that patients in hospitals often feel very stressed. It is perhaps easy to recognise this if we think about patients who are about to undergo major surgery, or have a life threatening illness. However, people who are in hospital for what we might regard as relatively minor complaints are also likely to feel stressed.

One of the main reasons is their feeling of uncertainty about what is going to happen next. Because we are familiar with our work environment we sometimes forget that to our patients the hospital or clinic is a strange and disturbing place.

Accounts by patients in hospital show that lack of communication is a major theme. As a care assistant you may have far more conversation with the patient than senior staff. You are therefore in a unique position to put patients at ease.

On admission, if the patient can go with you, you can show them the layout of the ward, explain the ward routine and how to recognise the different types of staff. You may sometimes be put in a difficult position when patients ask you about their medical condition or nursing treatment. If this does happen it is important that you pass this information on to the nurse in charge of the ward, or if appropriate the patient's "named nurse", who will deal with the enquiry.

A very interesting development in recent years has been the introduction of complementary therapies on hospital wards. Massage and aromatherapy have been found especially useful in relieving patients' stress.

Women and stress

The majority of care assistants are women, and as a group may have additional causes of stress not experienced by their male colleagues.

Child care

Women with children may have particular problems. These may include practical difficulties of fitting in work hours around their children. Problems may also arise because of the economic necessity of working, while feeling guilty about leaving children in the care of other people. Financial pressures may also be evident because of the high cost of childminders and nursery placements.

There are no easy solutions to these difficulties. It is important that when you are experiencing problems you discuss them – possibly with your manager. The majority of nurse managers are sympathetic and may have experienced similar problems themselves. Employers are becoming more enlightened in their approach and some are offering workplace creches, and also job share schemes.

Sexual harassment

Another recently identified cause of stress in the workplace, predominantly experienced by women, is sexual harassment. Sexual harassment includes unwanted physical contact, offensive flirtations, constantly being asked out, unwelcome, sexist and patronising language, and sexual assault.

Dealing with these situations is difficult. If harassment occurs it should be reported to a senior person immediately. You may wish to seek advice from other people – possibly from your union representative.

Points to remember

1. Stress is a response to threat.
2. It is generally recognised that hospitals are stressful environments.
3. Key life events have been identified as being stressful.
4. You will have physical symptoms if you are experiencing stress.
5. An important way to deal with stress is to talk to someone you can trust.
6. Try to identify stressful parts of your life, and if possible remove the cause or seek ways to deal with the problem.
7. Poor communication is a major cause of stress to hospital patients.
8. If bad practice is witnessed it must be reported to a senior person.
9. Sexual harassment should not be tolerated in the workplace.
10. Stress can be a beneficial experience if successfully overcome.

NVQ Levels 2 & 3 Value Base Units

Ob Maintain confidentiality of information.
Oe Support individuals through effective communication.

Levels 2 & 3 Core Units

U4 Contribute to the health, safety and security of individuals and their care environment. *Particularly* U4d Maintain personal standards of health safety and security.
U5 Obtain, transmit and store information relating to the delivery of a care service.

CHAPTER 22

Further training and opportunities

Lynne Swiatczak

*• Changing and developing roles for care assistants • Courses within the hospital
• Vocational training and qualifications • College courses • Open learning
• Entry into nurse training*

Some people find the role of the care assistant fulfilling and are happy to remain in that role in a particular area. Others feel that they would like to develop further either in their present role or by applying for other posts.

There are many opportunities for care assistants, particularly since the introduction of National Vocational Qualifications (NVQs) - see Chapter 23. New roles and specialised jobs have evolved, and are developing still.

Some hospitals have created new roles which allow for specialism in certain areas for example some accident and emergency departments employ care assistants to carry out diagnostic tests such as ECGs (electrocardiographs). Other areas have created roles which extend the care assistant role into more traditional nursing duties – dressing wounds, taking observations, etc. There are also opportunities to move into other disciplines, for example physiotherapy helper, occupational therapy aide or social work assistant.

Each individual must decide what it is they wish to do, and in order to do this

they must collect as much information as they can about courses and other training opportunities.

There are several ways of obtaining information:
• Your ward sister/charge nurse may have access to training and development programmes within your hospital.
• Local colleges have information on courses available.
• Nursing journals such as *Elderly Care* and *Paediatric Nursing* often carry articles which are specifically for care assistants, and this is a useful way of keeping up to date in your area.

Within the hospital

Many hospitals provide specific training and development for their unqualified staff. This can range from basic induction courses to specific courses in various special areas, for example elderly care, paediatric care and surgical care.

Some of these courses provide a certificate of attendance and completion which can be used to show prospective employers that a course has been undertaken.

These courses enable the care assistant to develop further knowledge and skills in the area in which they work, and also give a "taste" of training which can help staff decide whether to take other courses.

There are also specific courses such as First Aid at Work and Basic Resuscitation skills which are usually available to all staff.

Other courses may be available in areas such as assertiveness training, complementary therapies and massage. These courses are usually available to all staff and can provide a way of expanding your role without substantially changing it.

NVQs and SVQs

National Vocational Qualifications and Scottish Vocational Qualifications (SVQs or "Scotvecs") have ben developed as a national system of work-based qualifications (see Chapter 23). These qualifications are recognised nationally and are transferable between employers.

College courses

Many colleges offer courses in caring skills, ranging from short courses to certificate and diploma level. They each publish a prospectus for the academic year and this is available from the colleges and also from local libraries.

The Business and Technology Education Council (BTEC) awards many types of certificates and diplomas throughout the country. The courses offered in the area of care are many and varied. Some are full time and some part time, enabling staff to study in their own time. BTEC courses range

from Certificates in Social Care and Access to Nursing courses, to Diplomas in Science and Health Care. There are also **City and Guilds** courses and awards, similar in content and worth to BTEC courses. Details of these courses are also available from local colleges. Both BTEC and City and Guilds are awarding bodies for NVQs.

Open learning

The Open University, the Open College and many other organisations now provide open learning courses. These rely on the dedication and enthusiasm of the student as there is little formal teaching. A tutor is usually appointed who may provide one-to-one tutorials. Much of the resource material is in book form although tapes and TV are also used. There are a variety of courses available in this format and they allow for flexibility of study. The main drawback to these courses is that there is often little group support.

The **Open University** provides a wide range of courses related to care professions. There are short courses with little assessed work, courses which involve assignments and courses which can lead to diploma and degree levels which have assignments and examinations.

The Open University requires self-motivation although you are allocated a tutor for support and often there are group meetings and seminars available. This is another flexible method of study, although some of the courses are quite expensive. Many care assistants/health care support workers find this method of study fits in with family commitments and also enables them to remain in the clinical area.

The **Open College** also offers flexible training packages in Health and Care, with self-study workbooks, study guides, audio cassettes and assignment material. The packages include guidelines for your manager so that support can be given by staff in your workplace.

Nurse training

Many care assistants/health care support workers decide that they wish to apply for nurse training. The role of care assistant allows them to experience the hospital environment and to observe the different role of the nurse. If this option is decided upon then there is usually a need to complete some training or an access course before commencing nurse education.

In recent years colleges of nursing have developed **Project 2000**, a new form of nurse training. This removes some of the apprentice-type training of the past. Project 2000 training is more theoretical in nature, then this theory is applied this to nursing practice. Student nurses are students; they are not expected to be a "pair of hands" on the wards. It is also at a higher academic level, and nurses who qualify in Project 2000 gain the Diploma in Nursing together with their nursing qualification.

The training also stresses the importance of seeing each individual as a whole person rather than a collection of illnesses. Students complete the same foundation training and then split into "branches". These are adult, paediatric, mental health, learning disability and specific training for midwifery.

The entry requirements vary although five GCSE Levels or equivalent is usually the norm. Some colleges allow access via a special entrance test and other access courses. These are particularly useful for mature entrants. The qualifications above are the minimum accepted and as the course is academically demanding care assistants must be sure that this is what they wish to do. If you are interested in nurse training you should contact your local college of nursing for initial details and then apply via the UKCC clearing house (the UKCC is the nurses' governing body).

There are also several courses available in hospitals and colleges which look at assertiveness, self-awareness and counselling skills. Some areas, such as mental health and elderly care, often require care assistants to be skilled in these areas and provide relevant courses. Other care assistants may like to undertake these courses in their own time at local colleges. They are very beneficial as they encourage the care assistant to have insight into their own strengths and needs, and often provide the impetus to move on to other types of training.

Addresses

BTEC, Central House, Upper Woburn Place, London WC1H 0HH. Tel: 071 413 8400.

City and Guilds, 46 Brittania Street, London WC1X 9RG. Tel: 071 278 2468.

The Open College, St Paul's, 781 Wilmslow Road, Didsbury, Greater Manchester M20 8RW.

Open University, Information Office, Department of Health and Social Welfare, Milton Keynes, MK7 6AA. Tel: 0908 653743.

National Council for Vocational Qualifications (NCVQ), 222 Euston Road, London NW1 2BZ. Tel: 071 387 9898.

Joint Awarding Body, 46 Britannia St, London WC1X 9RG. Tel: 071 278 2468. *Information on the NVQ care standards and your nearest assessment centre.*

Nurses and Midwives Central Clearing House, PO Box 346, Bristol BS99 7FB.

CHAPTER 23

National Vocational Qualifications

by Judith Roberts

What are NVQs and what use are they to you? • The way training and assessment works • How you can get started

National Vocational Qualifications (NVQs) are a country wide system of qualifications related to job skills and occupations. In Scotland they are called Scottish Vocational Qualifications (SVQs). NVQs/SVQs apply not only to the care sector, but are also available in many other fields of work, from horse grooming to hairdressing, motor vehicle repair to management.

All NVQ awards are based on the idea of competence – the ability to perform in the workplace, to the standards that the occupation requires.

An NVQ is gained when the candidate is assessed performing in a real work situation, doing a real job, to the required standards. But skills on their own are not enough. The worker has to show that they understand why they are doing the task in that way; in other words some "underpinning knowledge" is necessary.

The benefits of NVQs

• NVQs allow you to build up parts of the award, or "credits", gradually. It doesn't matter when you do them or how long it takes. This helps people fit in training around domestic or work commitments.

• There is open access: anyone can apply to be assessed.

• Assessment can be obtained and achieved independently of the time or methods of any accompanying learning. Distance or Open Learning becomes a practical solution for people who work unsocial hours.

• NVQs do not demand time away from the workplace, and their development and the assessment process is directly relevant and meaningful to the worker.

• It is learning by doing, an active process that for many people makes the learning process more enjoyable, more relevant and more effective.

Why get involved?

Candidates who have achieved NVQ awards in Care have said that the process of becoming qualified has meant:

• They are more aware of their clients' needs and rights, especially their emotional, social and cultural needs.

• They feel they now give more individualised care, and are more useful to other members of the team.

• They are now more aware of the "How?" and "Why?" of their practice, and are able to describe their experience using a more "professional" vocabulary.

• They consider themselves to be better informed, more assertive and confident, and better able to challenge inadequate practice.

• They found the support and recognition offered to them by their work based assessor valuable, and often developed more effective working relations with others.

Standards have been decided on, after years of work developing and testing them, by representatives from each field of work, called Lead Industry Bodies (LIB). The LIB for the care sector is the Care Sector Consortium.

NVQs are awarded by organisations called Awarding Bodies. Examples are City and Guilds and the Central Council for Education and Training in Social Work (CCETSW).

Levels of awards

All NVQs are graded, rising from Level 1 to Level 5. The higher the Level, the greater the breadth and complexity of the qualification. This allows the worker to progress within the qualification structure as their skills, knowledge and respon-sibilities increase and broaden.

Level 1 Foundation and basic work activities

Level 2 A broad range of skills and responsibilities

Level 3 Complex/skilled and/or supervisory work

Level 4 Managerial/specialist

Level 5 Professional/senior managerial

The NVQ framework

NVQ awards have a common structure. Each different Level is made up of a number of Units. These Units are in turn split into several Elements of Competence.

Each Element contains "performance criteria" (details of what is expected of you as you perform the task), "range statements" where you need to show competence in a range of care situations, and details of the "underpinning knowledge" you are required to show.

Taking one Element at a time, the worker is assessed working in each of the situations specified in the Element. Their standard of competence is assessed against the performance criteria and underpinning knowledge that Element requires. Through this process the worker can slowly build up their qualification. This is called "credit accumulation".

NVQs Awards in Care: the Integrated Standards

NVQs in both social care and nursing settings have been brought together, and there are qualifications available at Levels 2 and 3. These awards give care workers more choice and opportunity for progression in jobs across both sectors, and represent more closely the wide range of client groups, roles and responsibilities.

To the structure of Units and Elements described before, Endorsements are added. These are Units grouped together because they relate to the specific role of the candidate.

For example, care assistants working with elderly people need some of the same skills and knowledge, and some different skills and knowledge, from care assistants working in postnatal departments. So both will work through the same Core Units as described earlier, plus the Endorsement for their work area.

People involved in the assessment process

A *candidate* is the worker being assessed for an NVQ.

A *work based assessor* (WBA) is the person who carries out the assessment of the candidate. The WBA is usually a more senior colleague who has a broad expertise in the work. Increasingly it is expected that the assessor will also have proved they are competent to assess the work of others.

The WBA's assessment decisions are checked by a person called the *Internal Verifier* (IV) whose role is to make sure that the assessments carried out by the WBA meet the NVQ standards and the Awarding Body assessment requirements. This person should come from a different work setting or section from the WBA.

How to start

There are three main processes involved:
1. Collect information so that you can see which Levels and Endorsements would be best for you.
2. Identify your training requirements and how you can obtain any necessary training.
3. Find out how, and by whom, you can be assessed in the workplace. It is likely that your training section or school of nursing is already an assessment centre.

Remember, without the opportunity for assessment, and verification of the assessment, you will not get your qualification.

1. Information gathering

You will need to find out:
• Is your workplace considering getting involved with NVQs? Whom should you contact, where and when? This is not always easy if you work nights or weekends, but persevere. It is likely that other care assistants, the ward sister or manager, or your union, will know more.
• More information about NVQs, and especially about NVQs in Care. This information should be available from your training department, but it also could be obtained from the Career Service, the local Training and Enterprise Council (TEC), the National Council for Vocational Qualifications, your union or local colleges.
• Which level of award and choice of endorsement would be appropriate for you? This will be decided in discussion with your immediate line manager and the training centre.
• What existing knowledge could you be accredited with, and what additional training might you require?
• When are you likely to be accepted onto an NVQ programme and offered assessment? There may be some delay, so it could be useful to see if there are any appropriate programmes or short courses you could attend while waiting. Accreditation of Prior Learning should be available, so this would not be wasted.
• What costs, if any, might you have to pay towards your assessment? Ask whether your local TEC is sponsoring NVQs, especially if there is any financial support.
• Where will any training occur? Will you have to do it in your own time? Is attendance at the training sessions compulsory?
• How quickly will they expect you to complete all your assessments? (Less than three months is unrealistic unless you and your assessor are very committed and your ward not too busy.)
• Is there open access? Do you have to be employed for a certain length of time? Will they only assess day staff? (They shouldn't – this could contravene their equal opportunities policy.)
• Do you have to be recommended by your line manager?
• Will they expect you to stay in employment for a stated length of time following completion – or pay any fees back?
• Will you be allowed to progress to the Level 3 qualification? (As yet the use of Level 3 NVQ in Care as an entry qualification for student nurse education has to be resolved, but if this is of any interest to you, contact your local School of Nursing to find out more.)

2. Undertake any training required

This could be through a variety of routes and take varying lengths of time. It is recommended that for a Level 2 award training should take between six and ten

NATIONAL VOCATIONAL QUALIFICATIONS

months, and for a Level 3 award about one year. Obviously it depends on your previous knowledge, and how recently any training took place. When enquiring about your training, find answers to the following questions:
• Does your workplace offer training on site or do you have to go elsewhere for it?
• How many actual hours of tuition will you receive? How big are the classes?
• Is there access to a library? Are any other resources available?
• What methods will be used to deliver the "underpinning knowledge"? Will any specialists be teaching you? How much tutorial support will you be offered?

3. Getting assessed in the workplace

This will depend upon the policy of your employer. You should be able to find out who is to be your assesssor, so make time to get to know them (although it will probably be someone you have already worked with).

Don't forget that at first both you and your assessor may be anxious or uncertain. You may have to develop a working relationship that suits you both.

The "Standards" may look like a foreign language, but after time and lots of reading they do become more "user-friendly". So once you are given the Standards, do start to read them. Ask if you do not understand a word or phrase – others are probably wondering too!

Start taking notice of your practice and the practice of others, reflect on what you observe and discuss it if you can with your assessor or tutor. Trust yourself: you may have things to learn, but don't forget you are already doing the job. You probably know more than you think.

Finally the work of the Internal Verifier is checked by an *External Verifier*, who is appointed by the Awarding Body and has no connection with your hospital or workplace.

Your assessment

The assessment methods are designed to be flexible and easily organised, with the assessment timetable being devised and controlled by the candidate. This is called "Assessment on demand".

The commonest method of assessment, particularly in care, is assessment by direct observation of the candidate's work. However, another eight methods are also acceptable, These can include simulations (role playing), oral or written questions, assignments, completion of work products such as reports or records, or testimony of others (clients, other workers).

A typical assessment might run as follows:

1 A worker checks the assessment requirements of the element. They check to see if they have sufficient underpinning knowledge and skills. They may ask the opinion of an impartial adviser to help decide this. They may decide to undertake training or support. The training could be "in house", from a more senior colleague or training officer, or from a planned course or programme, which may or may not be achieved through Open or Distance Learning.

2 Following training the candidate checks that they now have the required knowledge and skills, that they now feel confident in their ability and are ready for assessment.

3 The candidate approaches their WBA, and requests assessment. The assessor talks about the impending assessment, checks the candidate is fully aware of the assessment requirements, and might offer to do a "practice assessment". They will

discuss any queries, and only when they *both* feel confident that the worker is ready to be assessed will they arrange a date that suits them both.

In the case of the care awards, they also approach a suitable client or clients, to ask if they would agree to be involved. It is vitally important that the client gives informed consent, and is not coerced in any way. If a client is confused or has limited understanding, the family should be asked for permission if at all possible.

4 The assessment day. The candidate will confirm with the client that they are still happy to be involved and the assessor will confirm that the candidate is ready. Throughout whatever activity is taking place the assessor will observe the candidate, as unobtrusively as is practical.

After the observation of the candidate's practice the assessor will question the candidate, and may ask to see any relevant documentation or reports. This helps the WBA to check on any aspects of the assessment process and helps to make sure that the candidate has the understanding and knowledge specified in the standards. Then, and only then, will the assessor confirm to the candidate their decision: either the candidate is competent or not yet competent.

Once the decision has been recorded, the assessor will explain to the candidate, in as much detail as is required, why they made that decision, if necessary giving comments or advice that will help the candidate improve their practice in future.

At the end of the process they will make an appointment for the assessment of a new element, or if necessary a re-assessment. All necessary documentation is completed and made available for the Internal Verifier to see.

5 Once the assessor has completed a few assessments the IV will be invited to check on the documentation and the candidates' records of evidence.

6 Finally when all the units of the award have been assessed and the candidate is declared competent, the External Verifier will be invited to visit the assessment centre to view the assessment records (probably those of other candidates as well). They will make their decision based upon the evidence they check. Once the assessments have External Verifier approval the candidates will receive their qualification certificates.

Awards in Care
NVQs/SVQs Level 2

Level 2 Core
O Promote equality for all individuals
Z1 Contribute to the protection of individuals from abuse
W2 Contribute to the ongoing support of clients and others significant to them
W3 Support clients in transition due to their care requirements
U4 Contribute to the health, safety and security of individuals and their environment
U5 Obtain, transmit and store information relating to the delivery of a care service

Direct Care Endorsement
Z6 Enable clients to maintain and improve their mobility
Z7 Contribute to the movement and treatment of clients to maximise their physical comfort
Z9 Enable clients to maintain their personal hygiene and appearance
Z10 Enable clients to eat and drink
Z11 Enable clients to access and use toilet facilities
Z19 Enable clients to achieve physical comfort

These are the Units you need to work through to achieve NVQ Level 2 in Care with the Direct Care Endorsement.

See page 144 for useful addresses.

Useful addresses

All these organisations welcome a stamped, self-addressed envelope sent with your enquiry.

Action for Dysphasic Adults, Canterbury House, 1 Royal Street, London SE1 7LN. Tel: 071 261 9572.

Action for Victims of Medical Accidents, Bank Chambers, 1 London Road, Forest Hill, London SE23 3TP. Tel: 081 291 2793.

Afro Caribbean Mental Health Association, 35-37 Electric Avenue, Brixton, London SW9 8JP. 071 737 3603.

Afro Caribbean Society for the Blind, 12 Lilac Gardens, Shirley, Surrey CR0 8NR.

Age Concern England, Astral House, 1268 London Road, London SW16 4ER. Tel: 081 679 8000.

Age Exchange Reminiscence Centre, 11 Blackheath Village, London SE3 9LA. Tel: 081 318 9105.

AIDS Helpline, National. Tel: 0800 567 123. Ethnic minority language lines also available.

Alcohol Concern, 275 Grays Inn Road, London WC1. Tel: 071 833 3471.

Alzheimer's Disease Society, Gordon House, 10 Greencoat Place London SW1P 1PH. Tel: 071 306 0606.

Arthritis Care, 5 Grosvenor Crescent, London SW1X 7ER. Tel: 071 235 0902.

ASBAH (Association for Spina Bifida and Hydrocephalus), Asbah House, 42 Park Road, Peterborough PE1 2UQ. Tel: 0733 555988.

Asian People's Disability Alliance, Ground Floor, Willesden Hospital, Harlesden Rd, London NW10. Tel: 081 459 5793.

Association of Blind Asians, 322 Upper St, London N1 2XQ. Tel: 071 226 1950.

Association of Continence Advisers, at the Disabled Living Foundation, 380-384 Harrow Road, London W9 2HU. Tel: 071 289 6111.

Breast Care and Mastectomy Association of Great Britain, 15-19 Britten St, London SW3 3TZ. 071 867 8275. Helpline 071 867 1103.

British Assoctiation of Cancer United Patients BACUP), 3 Bath Place, London EC2A 3JR. Tel.: 071 696 9003.

British Association of the Hard of Hearing, 7-11 Armstrong Road, London W3 7JL. Tel: 081 743 1110.

British Association of Occupational Therapists, 6-8 Marshalsea Rd, Southwark, London SE1 1HL. Tel: 071 357 6480.

British Colostomy Association, 38-39 Eccleston Square, London SW1V 1PB. Tel: 071 828 5175.

British Complementary Medicine Association, Exmoor Street, London W10 6DZ. Tel: 081 964 1205.

British Deaf Association, 38 Victoria Place, Carlisle. Tel: 0228 48844.

British Diabetic Association, 10 Queen Anne Street, London W1M 0BD. 071 323 1531.

British Epilepsy Association, Anstey House, 40 Hanover Square, Leeds LS3 1BE. Tel: 0532 439393.

(local call charge only).

British Heart Foundation , 14 Fitxhardinge St, London W1H 4DH. Tel: 071 935 0185.

British Institute of Learning Disabilities, Information and Resource Centre, Wolverhampton Rd, Kidderminster, Worcs DY10 3PP. Tel: 0562 850251.

British Kidney Patient Association, Bordon, Hampshire GU35 9JZ. Tel: 0420 472 021/2.

British Pregnancy Advisory Service, Austy Manor, Wootton Wawen, Solihull, West Midlands B95 6BX. Tel: 0564 793225.

British Red Cross Society, 9 Grosvenor Crescent, London SW1X 7EJ. Tel: 071 235 5454. Volunteer beauty care and other services.

Brittle Bone Society, 112 City Road, Dundee DD2 2PW. Tel: 0382 67603.

BTEC (Business and Technology Education Council) Central House, Upper Woburn Place, London WC1H 0HH. Tel: 071 413 8400.

Cancer Care Society, 21 Zetland Rd, Redland, Bristol BS6 7AH. Tel: 0272 427 419/232302.

Cancer Relief Macmillan Fund 15-19 Britten St, London SW3 3TZ. Tel: 071 351 7811.

Carers National Association, 29 Chilworth Mews, London W2 3RG. Tel: 071 724 7776.

Central Council for Education and Training in Social Work (CCETSW), Derbyshire

House, St Chad Street, London WC1H 8AD. Tel: 071 278 2455.

Centre for Policy on Ageing, 25-31 Ironmonger Row, London EC1V 3QP. Tel: 071 253 1787.

Chartered Society of Physiotherapy, 14 Bedford Row, London WC1. Tel: 071 242 1941.

Chest, Heart and Stroke Association, CHSA House, 123-127 Whitecross St, London EC1Y 8JJ. Tel: 071 490 7999.

Chinese Mental Health Association, c/o Working World Trust, Unit 20, Peterley Business Centre, 472 Hackney Road, London E2 9EQ. 071 613 1008.

Christian Council on Ageing, The Old Court, Greens Norton, Nr Towcester, Northants NN12 8BS. Tel: 0327 50481.

City and Guilds, 46 Brittania Street, London WC1X 9RG. Tel: 071 278 2468.

College of Speech and Language Therapists, Lechmere Rd, London NW2 5BU.

Commission for Racial Equality, Eliot House, Arlington St, London SW1. Tel: 071 828 7022.

Counsel and Care for the Elderly, Twyman House, 16 Bonny Street, London NW1 9PG. Tel: 071 485 1550.

Cruse – Bereavement Care, Cruse House, 126 Sheen Road, Richmond, Surrey TW9 1UR. Tel: 081 940 4818.

Cystic Fibrosis Trust, Alexandra House, 5 Blythe Rd, Bromley, Kent BR1 3RS. Tel: 081 464 7211.

Disabled Living Foundation, 380-384 Harrow Road, London W9 2HU. Tel: 071 289 6111.

Down's Syndrome Association, 155 Mitcham Rd, London SW17 9PG. Tel: 081 682 4001.

Endometriosis Society, 35 Belgrave Square, London SW1 8PQ. Tel: 071 235 4136/7.

Equal Opportunities Commission, Overseas House, Quay St, Manchester M3 3HN. Tel: 061 833 9244.

Friedreich's Ataxia Group, Copse Edge, Thursley Rd, Elstead, Godalming, Surrey GU8 6DJ. Tel: 0252 702 864.

Haemophilia Society, 123 Westminster Bridge Road, London SE1 7HR. Tel: 071 928 2020.

Headway (National Head Injuries Association Ltd) King Edward Court, 7 King Edward St, Nottingham. Tel: 0602 240800.

Help the Aged, 16-18 St James's Walk, Clerkenwell, London EC1R 0BE. Tel: 071 253 0253.

Huntingdon's Disease (Association to Combat), 108 Battersea High St, London SW11 3HP. Tel: 071 223 7000.

Hysterectomy Support Network, 3 Lynne Close, Green Street Green, Orpington, Kent BR6 6BS. Tel: 081 856 3881.

Ileostomy Association, Amblehurst House, Black Scotch Lane, Mansfield, Notts NG18 4PF. Tel: 0623 28099.

Incontinence Advisory Service, The Disabled Living Foundation, 380-384 Harrow Rd, London W9 2HU. Tel: 071 289 6111.

International Cerebral Palsy Society, 5a Netherhall Gdns, London NW3 5RN. Tel: 071 794 9761.

Jewish Care, Stewart Young House, 221 Golders Green Road, London NW11 9DQ. Tel: 081 458 3282.

Laryngectomy Clubs (National Association), Ground Floor, 6 Rickett St, Fulham, London SW6 1RU. Tel: 071 381 9993.

Limbless Association, 31 The Mall, Ealing, London W5 2PX. Tel: 081 579 1758.

MENCAP, Royal Society for Mentally Handicapped Children and Adults, 123 Golden Lane, London EC1Y 0RT. Tel: 071 454 0454.

MIND/National Association for Mental Health, 22 Harley Street, London W1N 2ED. Tel: 071 637 0741.

Mobility Information Service, National Mobility Centre, Unit 2a. Atcham Industrial Estate, Shrewsbury SY4 4UG. Tel: 0743 761 889.

Motor Neurone Disease Association, PO Box 246, Northampton NN1 2PR. Tel: 0604 22269/250505. Helpline 0345 626262.

Multiple Sclerosis Society of Great Britain and Northern Ireland, 25 Effie Road, Fulham, London SW6 1EE. Tel: 071 736 6267.

Muscular Dystrophy Group, 7-11 Prescott Place, London SW4 6BS. Tel: 071 720 8055.

Myasthenia Gravis Association, Central Office, Keynes House, 77 Nottingham Road, Derby DE1 3QS. Tel: 0332 290219.

National Association for Colitis and Crohn's Disease, 98A London Rd, St Albans, Herts. AL1 1NX. Tel: 0727 844296.

National Autistic Society, 276 Willesden Lane, London NW2 5RB. Tel: 081 451 1114.

National Back Pain Association, 31-33 Park Rd, Teddington, Middx TW11 0AB. Tel: 081 977 5474.

National Childbirth Trust, Alexandra House, Oldham Terrace, Acton, London W3 6NH. Tel: 081 992 8637.

National Deaf-Blind and Rubella Association (SENSE), 11-13 Clifton Terrace, London N4. Tel: 071 278 1005.

National Deaf Blind League, 18 Rainbow Court, Paston Ridings, Peterborough PE4 6UP. Tel: 0733 73511.

National Meningitis Trust, Fern House, Bath Road, Stroud, Glos GL5 3TJ. Tel: 0453 751 738. Helpline 0453 755 049.

National Osteoporosis Society, PO Box 10, Radstock, Bath. BA3 3YB.

National Schizophrenia Fellowship, 28 Castle Street, Kingston-upon-Thames, Surrey KT1 1SS. Tel: 081 547 3937.

National Society for Epilepsy, Information Department, Chalfont St Peter, Buckinghamshire SL9 0RJ. Tel: 02407 3991.

National Toy Libraries Association, 68 Churchway, London NW1 1LT. 071 387 9592.

Nottingham Rehab Ltd, 17 Ludlow Hill Road, Melton Road, West Bridgford, Nottingham NG2 6HD. Tel: 0602 452345. A variety of activity materials and aids - catalogue available.

Open College, St Paul's, 781 Wilmslow Rd, Didsbury, Greater Manchester M20 8RW.

Open University, Information Office, Department of Health and Social Welfare, Milton Keynes MK7 6AA. Tel: 0908 653743.

Paget's Disease (National Association for the Relief of), Room B304, CSB Hope Hospital, Salford, Manchester. M6 8HD. Tel: 061 787 4949.

Pain Society, 9 Benford Square, London WC1B 3RA. Tel: 071 631 1650.

Parkinson's Disease Society of the UK. 22 Upper Woburn Place, London WC1H 0RA. Tel: 071 383 3513.

Patients Association, 18 Victoria Park Sqaure, Bethnal Green, London E2 9PF. Tel: 081 981 5676/5695.

Perthes Disease Association, 42 Woodland Road, Guildford, Surrey GU1 1RW. Tel: 0483 306637.

PHAB (Physically Handicapped and Able-Bodied together) 14 London Rd, Croydon CR0 2TA. Tel: 081 667 9443.

Phenylketonuria (National Society for), 7 Southfield Close, Willem, Milton Keynes MK15 9LL. Tel: 0908 691653.

QUIT (help to stop smoking), 102 Gloucester Place, London W1H 3DA. Tel: 071 487 2858. Quitline 071 487 3000.

Royal College of Nursing of the UK, 20 Cavendish Square, London W1M 0AB. Tel: 071 409 3333.

Royal National Institute for the Blind, 224 Great Portland Street, London W1N 6AA. Tel: 071 388 1266.

Royal National Institute for the Deaf, 105 Gower Street, London WC1E 6AH. Tel: 071 387 8033.

Sickle Cell and Thalassaemia Information Centre, St Leonard's Hospital, Nutall St, London N1 5LZ. Tel: 071 739 8484.

Social Care Association, 23a Victoria Rd, Surbiton, Surrey. Tel: 081 390 6831/4639.

Schizophrenia Association of Great Britain. Bryn Hyfryd, The Crescent, Bangor, Gwynedd LL57 2AG. Tel: 0248 354048.

Spinal Injuries Association, Newpoint House, 76 St James's Lane, London N10M 3DF. Tel: 081 444 2121. Helpline 081 883 4296.

SPOD (Sexual and personal relationships of disabled people) 286 Camden Rd, Lonbdon N7 0BJ. Tel: 071 607 8851.

Stillbirth and Neonatal Death Society (SANDS) 28 Portland Place London W1N 4DE. Tel: 071 436 5881.

Talking Books for the Handicapped (National Listening Library), 12 Lant Street, London SE1 1QR. Tel: 071 407 9417. A postal lending library service of literature recorded on long-playing cassettes.

TFH, 76 Barracks Road, Sandy Lane Industrial Estate, Stourport-on-Severn, Worcestershire DY13 9QB. Tel: 0299 827820. Games, puzzles, pastimes etc for disabled/older people.

Turner Syndrome Society, Child Growth Foundation, 2 Mayfield Avenue, London W4 1PW. Tel: 081 994 7625.

University of the Third Age, 1 Stockwell Green, SW9 9JF. Tel: 071 737 2541. Promotes and organises self-help educational activities for older people.

Winslow Press, Telford Road, Bicester, Oxfordshire OX6 0TS. Tel: 0869 244733. Books, activities, games, reminiscence materials.

Women's Health, 52-54 Featherstone St, London EC1Y 8RT. Tel: 071 251 6580. Information, resources and support.

Glossary of terms

Abdomen. The stomach or belly. This area of the body is described as extending from just under the rib cage down to the top of the thighs.

AIDS (Acquired Immunodeficiency Syndrome - see also HIV). AIDS is a condition caused by a virus called HIV (Human Immunodeficiency Virus). This damages the body's defence system so that it cannot fight infection. AIDS causes many people to develop certain forms of cancer, and to get serious infections of the lungs, digestive system, the brain and skin. It is passed on by exchanging body fluids such as blood, semen and vaginal fluids.

Alzheimer's disease (see also Dementia). A form of dementia characterised by changes to the brain, although the particular cause is unknown. Disorientation, loss of memory, loss of intellectual function, apathy and difficulty with coordinating movement, speech or thoughts, are common features.

Amnesia. Loss of memory.

Amputation. Accidental loss, or surgical removal, of a limb.

Anaemia. Shortage of the oxygen-carrying part (haemoglobin) of the blood's red cells. This may be because the body is losing too much haemoglobin (for example due to bleeding from the rectum), or because it is not making enough (for example due to a shortage of iron in the diet).

Anaesthetic. A substance that can cause temporary loss of the sensation of pain or consciousness. As a "local" anaesthetic it numbs a specific part of the body only. As a "general" anaesthetic it causes the patient to lose consciousness.

Analgesics. Medicines that provide relief from pain.

Angina. Chest pain due to oxygen shortage in the heart muscles. Caused by narrowing or blockage of the coronary arteries which supply the muscles with oxygen.

Antibiotics. Medicines which either kill bacteria or stop them multiplying and spreading. They have no effect on viruses.

Anti-convulsants. Medicines which are used to treat epilepsy.

Anus (see also Colon). The muscular ring at the end of the intestinal canal. The end of the pelvic colon.

Anxiety state. A condition in which the individual is so worried about a certain situation or problem, that their life is severely restricted. The main characteristic is the inability to relax.

Arteriosclerosis. A gradual loss of elasticity in the walls of arteries, due to thickening and the build up of calcium deposits. There is decreased blood flow and oxygen supply to essential parts of the brain and body.

Arthritis (see also Osteoarthritis and Rheumatoid arthritis). Inflammation causing pain, stiffness and swelling in one or more joints. There may be serious deformity (eg of the hands) and disability. There are several different types of arthritis, including osteoarthritis and rheumatoid arthritis. Main causes are inflammation, and the effects of wear and tear.

Aseptic. Free from living disease-causing organisms.

Asthma. A condition in which the tubes of the lung have a fluctuating and reversible tendency to narrow causing breathlessness, coughing, wheezing or chest tightness. The triggers to this narrowing may be allergens such as house dust mite, animal fur, pollens or something quite different like infections, fumes, smoke, cold air or exercise. Some people are sensitive to certain medicines, food colourings or alcohol.

Antiseptic. A substance opposing sepsis (infection) by arresting the growth of microorganisms.

Autopsy. See post mortem.

Behaviour modification. A programme in which a specific goal or reward is provided to correct an inappropriate behaviour. It is repeatedly reinforced over a period of days or weeks. Screaming or shouting may be lessened, for example, by providing regular individual attention when the person is not shouting or screaming.

Blood pressure (see also Hypertension). The force of blood in the arteries measured in millimetres of mercury by a machine called a sphygmomanometer. Blood pressures are written down as two figures. The top figure is called the "systolic" and the bottom figure is known as the "diastolic". How high or low blood pressure is depends on the strength of the heart beat and the condition of the arteries.

Benign. When describing a tumour this means favourable, non-cancerous, usually contained within a capsule and not spreading to other parts of the body.

Bradycardia. A marked slowing of the rate of the heart.

Braille. A system of writing and printing by means of raised points representing letters which allows blind people to read by touch. From Louis Braille (1809-1852), a French teacher of blind people.

Bronchitis. Inflammation of the air tubes of the lungs. This may be "acute" due to a bacterial or viral infection. Or it may be "chronic" due to excessive production of mucus caused by many factors including pollution or smoking.

Bruising. The discolouration of skin which results from leakage of blood from a blood vessel, usually due to trauma.

Burn-out (see also Stress). A reaction to stress which may take various forms. The individual becomes unable to cope with all the physical and emotional demands made upon them.

Cancer. A large group of diseases which are linked together because in each case there is uncontrolled tissue growth of the affected part of the body. This tissue growth is always abnormal, may spread into organs nearby or far away (e.g. by blood or lymph spread to lymph glands, lung or brain) and may cause death. The outlook (prognosis) for each sufferer is very different depending on the site and type of their cancer.

Capillaries. The tiny blood vessels which lie between arteries bringing blood to the tissues and veins taking it away.

Cataract. A clouding of the lens of the eye which prevents light passing through it easily, making vision dim and sometimes lost altogether.

Catheter. A tube which is passed into the body to drain fluids from or inject fluids into an organ. The most common is the urinary catheter for draining the bladder.

Cerebral palsy. Permanent and usually non-progressive damage to the brain before, during or soon after birth, resulting in some loss of use of limbs, with or without mental defect.

Cerebrovascular accident (CVA). See Stroke.

Chemotherapy. The treatment of disease by medicines or chemicals. Often used in the context of treating cancer.

Chorea. Strange, uncoordinated movements of the body particularly limbs. See also Huntingdon's Chorea.

Chronic. A term used to describe a long-standing and continuing disease process marked by progressive deterioration (sometimes despite treatment).

Circumcision. An operation to remove all or part of the foreskin of the penis.

Cleft palate. Congenital failure of the two halves of the roof of the mouth to join together. Often found with hare lip, the failure of proper development of the upper lip.

Colon (see also Anus). A part of the large intestine that absorbs nutrients and fluid from the diet. It ends at the anus.

Concussion. Brief loss of consciousness produced by a knock to the head. The person becomes very pale, has a feeble pulse and shallow breathing.

Conjunctivitis. Inflammation of the white of the eye caused by a bacterial or viral infection, or by an allergy.

Constipation. Incomplete or infrequent action of the bowels, due to lack of muscle activity, insufficient fluids or inadequate diet.

Continence (see also Incontinence). The ability to control the functions of passing urine or faeces when desired.

Coronary artery disease. Narrowing or blockage of the arteries supplying the heart with oxygen. Usually due to atheroma, a fatty coating of the inner lining of the arteries. Also known as coronary heart disease (CHD).

Coronary heart disease (CHD). See Coronary artery disease.

Cramp. Muscular spasm of a muscle usually due to lack of oxygen reaching it.

CVA (Cerebrovascular accident). See Stroke.

Defaecation. The act of opening the bowels.

Dehydration. Excessive loss of fluid from the body caused by vomiting, diarrhoea or sweating, or because of inadequate fluid intake.

Dementia (see also Alzheimer's disease). An organic mental illness caused by changes to the brain. This may be a result of disease or damage. The principal changes include inability to learn and retain information, inability to recall recent events, and feelings of anxiety and depression. This leads to disorientation and confused behaviour.

Depression. A morbid sadness which is distinct from that which normally accompanies bereavement or loss. Its features include reduced enjoyment, slowness and a lack of interest in life or the lives of others.

Diabetes. Failure of the pancreas in the body to produce insulin, or failure of the body to use the insulin sufficiently. Insulin breaks down sugary foods, allowing the body to use them for energy. Diabetes results in too much sugar circulating in the blood. Normal body functioning, for example wound healing, is affected by the condition.

Disorientation. A state of confusion in which an individual has lost a sense of where they are, what time it is and what they are doing.

Diuretic. Medicine which stimulates the kidneys to produce more urine. Commonly used for the treatment of heart failure.

Diverticulitis. A condition in which there is inflammation of small pockets (diverticulae) of large bowel which stick through the muscle surrounding the bowel at weak points. Generally caused by long-standing constipation.

Dysarthria. Difficulty with articulating words, often due to a stroke.

Dysphasia. Difficulty speaking, particularly arranging words in an understandable way. Aphasia is inability to speak.

Encephalitis. Inflammation of the brain, usually due to a virus.

Enuresis (nocturnal). Bed-wetting.

Epilepsy. A condition in which disorganised electrical activity in the brain causes fits. These may involve the whole body, known as "grand mal" fits, or they may be less serious involving perhaps a short loss of full consciousness known as "petit mal" fits, or they may be confined to one part of the body (eg leg or arm) known as focal fits.

Faeces. Waste matter that is indigestible such as cellulose food (fibre), excreted by the bowel.

Fetus/foetus. The unborn child.

Fainting. A temporary loss of consciousness due to a fall in blood pressure. The person usually falls to the floor, as this is the way in which the body attempts to help the blood circulation, so that more oxygen can reach the brain.

Fracture. A broken bone. The signs and symptoms include pain, swelling, loss of power and shortening of the affected limb. A fracture at the point where the thigh bone is connected to the hip usually results in the limb being turned to the side.

Fibre (in diet). The term is used to describe food that is high in roughage, indigestible, which stimulates the action of the intestine.

Genital. Relating to the sexual organs of the man or woman.

Gangrene. Death and destruction of a part of the body (eg a toe) following the loss of the blood supply to it.

Guarding. A defensive action that a person may take to safeguard themselves or to prevent any pain. Also, specific surgical term to indicate extreme tenderness of the abdomen.

Glaucoma. An illness in which abnormally high fluid pressure inside the eye can damage it permanently.

Heart attack. Damage to an area of heart muscle (see infarct) due to obstruction of the artery supplying this area with blood. The main symptom is usually sudden severe chest pain. It may be accompanied by shock and an abnormal pulse rate (either very fast, irregular or slow). If the damaged area is large, the person may die. If it is less extensive the person will survive and the heart gradually recover.

Heart failure. The failure by the heart to perform its function of pumping blood round the body efficiently. The most common symptoms are breathlessness on minimal exertion, tiredness and swollen ankles.

Hemiplegia. Paralysis of one side of the body as a result of injury or disease of the brain or spinal cord. Most commonly due to stroke.

Hernia. Protrusion of an organ from its normal position in the body into another. The most common is the inguinal hernia in which bowel pushes through defects in the muscle of the groin. Also known as a "rupture".

Herpes zoster. The virus which causes the painful skin condition shingles.

HIV (Human Immunodeficiency Virus). The virus that causes AIDS. It is not one virus, but a family of many similar viruses. It weakens the body's defence system by entering and destroying white cells that normally protect the body from infection.

Huntington's chorea. A chronic disease that is passed on through family heredity. The mental and physical powers of the person are affected, leading to a type of dementia. It is usually characterised by profound stiffness, rigidity, and difficulty with speech and swallowing.

Hydrocephalus. Accumulation of cerebro-spinal fluid in and around the brain.

Hypertension. Raised blood pressure.

Hypotension. Low blood pressure.

Hypothermia. Body temperature abnormally below the usual value of 37 degrees centigrade. At about 35 degrees centigrade confusion and listlessness may begin, below 33 degrees centigrade the breathing and pulse rate and blood pressure may start to fall. If prolonged death may occur.

Incontinence (see also Continence). Inability to retain faeces or urine until a suitable time and place is found for their release.

Infarct. An area of the body which is damaged or dies as a result of not receiving enough oxygen from its arteries. This supply failure is usually due to a blockage of or haemorrhage from the artery. Frequently used as 'coronary' or 'myocardial' infarct to describe the damage done to heart muscle after a heart attack.

Insomnia. Difficulty getting to sleep or remaining asleep for long.

Intoxication (see also Toxin). Poisoning by drugs or harmful substances. This may also include a state of drunkenness produced by too much alcohol.

Intractable. Used to describe any condition that is difficult to control or cure.

Lumbago. Pain in the low back.

Malabsorption. The failure of the normal absorption by the gut of some or all of the contents of food. This can cause symptoms of malnutrition such as failure to grow (children), loss of weight, diarrhoea, or anaemia.

Malignant. Of a tumour, cancerous.

Medication (see also Sedation and Tranquilliser). Used to describe tablets, liquids or injections that are used to improve a person's physical or mental condition.

Meningitis. A serious infection of the tissues surrounding the brain.

Metabolism. The process of life. The need, for example, to eat, drink and sleep, and for the body to use the food and fluids to continue to work and repair tissue damage when required.

Melaena. The production of black, tarry stools containing blood from the upper part of the gut.

Metastasis. A secondary tumour which has spread by blood or lymph from primary cancerous tumours. The commonest sites for metastases include glands, lung and bone.

Micturition. The act of emptying the bladder of urine.

Motor neurone disease. A disease in which there is progressive destruction, for reasons unknown, of some of the nerves responsible for stimulating muscles. This causes increasing weakness of groups of muscles, most notably those involved with breathing and swallowing.

Motor strength. Strength that permits action of the limbs and body to move about. This usually includes the muscle and connective tissue that make up the series of levers and pulleys within the body.

Multiple sclerosis. An often fluctuating, sometimes progressive, disease of the brain and spinal cord in which plaque replaces areas of normal nervous tissue. Depending on the site and extent of plaque this causes a range of symptoms including difficulties with co-ordination, incontinence and problems with vision and speech.

Muscular dystrophy. Group of muscle disorders which are usually congenital, become apparent in adolescence and are usually progressive.

Neoplasm. A tumour or growth.

Neurological. Relating to the body's brain and nerves.

Neurosis. Neuroses are common conditions whose symptoms include anxiety, phobias, compulsive states and hysterical reactions. The person's personality and understanding of their problem usually remain intact, although they often cannot help themselves.

Neuro-transmitters. Chemical substances which help to pass a signal down a nerve.

Oedema. Excessive collection of tissue fluid, often round the ankles or at the base of the spine.

Organic. Relating to a body organ. The term is used to describe a disease process that has a known physical cause. Dementia for example is a result of damage to the brain.

Osteoarthritis (see also Arthritis). A form of arthritis. It usually affects older people and larger joints. The cause is unknown but sufferers may be prone to more wear and tear of joints. There is destruction of the spongy pads (cartilage) between the bones, and formation of small bony outgrowths at the edges of the bone joints.

Paralysis. Loss of movement (but not sensation) in a muscle or group of muscles normally under the person's control. May be due to damage to the muscle itself or to its nerve supply.

Paraplegia. Paralysis of the lower part of the body usually due to a spinal injury.

Parkinsonism. Symptoms that are similar to Parkinson's disease: shaking or trembling, rhythmical muscular tremors, rigidity and a mask-like face that shows no emotion. Thumb and fore fingers may move in a "rolling" fashion. It can be caused by tranquillisers used to treat mental health problems.

Phobia. An irrational fear which is so strong that it interferes with day-to-day life.

Post mortem. After death. Also used as a noun to describe the process by which a pathologist investigates the cause of a person's death by examining all organs (autopsy).

Pneumonia. Inflammation of the lungs due to bacterial, viral or fungal infections.

Prolapse. The abnormal descent of any organ from its normal anatomical position. The most common organs to prolapse are the womb and bladder.

Pressure sore. An area of skin and underlying tissues which die as a result of pressure persistently preventing the flow of blood through its blood vessels (eg from lying in the same position for long periods). It causes an ulcer or sore to develop. Also known as a bed sore.

Prognosis. The outlook for a person with a disease, in terms of death and disability.

Prosthesis. Manufactured substitute for a part of the body (for example artificial leg, false teeth, breast prosthesis).

Pruritus. Itching.

Psychosis. Severe mental illness where the symptoms affect the whole person. They often lose touch with reality, have no insight into their condition, and act in a way which does not fit into acceptable patterns of life. The person's personality may be affected by delusions and hallucinations.

Pyrexia. Raised body temperature.

Reality orientation. The way in which older people with mental illness are helped to keep in touch with the world around them. This may be through the individual use of large clocks, signs on doors and newspapers. It can also be used in groups where older people are encouraged to participate in activities that remind them, for example, of where they are and the time of year.

Recovery position. The safest position in which to place a person who has had a serious accident or suffered a catastrophe like a heart attack or stroke. The purpose is to make sure the airway is kept open and fluids like vomit or blood can flow out of the mouth rather than down into the lungs. If a back injury is suspected only move the person if it is unquestionably life-saving and then as gently as possible because movement may make the back injury permanently worse.

Rehabilitation. The process by which a team of health workers restores a person who has had a serious illness to as near the health state he or she had before the illness.

Reminiscence therapy. This may involve active participation by individuals or groups, using past life events to understand the reasons for their mental health problems. Or it can be an activity session, using objects and photographs from the past.

Rheumatoid arthritis (see also Arthritis). A form of arthritis occurring in the small and large joints. It is usually characterised by chronic inflammation. Little is known about the cause.

Rheumatism. Term loosely applied in ordinary speech to any pain of unknown cause in the joints or muscles.

Sacrum. Part of the lower end of the spine.

Sedative (see also Medication and Tranquilliser). A drug which reduces excitement, anxiety and tension.

Senile dementia (see Dementia). Dementia occurring in old age.

Shock. Physical collapse resulting from impaired blood circulation to vital organs. Common causes include severe bleeding or a heart attack which prevents the heart pumping the blood effectively.

Sphincter. The ring of muscle which surrounds the opening of a hollow organ like the bladder and which controls the escape of the contents of the organ until a suitable time.

Spina bifida. A congenital disease in which there is a defect in the bones of the spine. This can be mild (spina bifida occulta) and cause no symptoms. However in more serious forms the spinal cord can be damaged causing paralysis of the legs and incontinence of urine and faeces, often accompanied by mental retardation and hydrocephalus.

Sprain. An injury to a ligament when the joint it is supporting is forced through a range of movement greater than normal, without dislocation or fracture.

Stress (see also Burn-out). The reaction, both physical and mental, to the demands made upon a person. Stress reactions occur when the individual is unable to cope with all the demands made upon them.

Stroke. A brain disorder of rapid onset, usually caused by a blockage in or haemorrhage (bleeding) from one of the main arteries of the brain. Speech and movement are most commonly affected but other functions may be damaged, depending upon which part of the brain is involved. Speed of recovery depends on the extent of the blockage or haemorrhage. Also known as a cerebrovascular accident (CVA).

Tachycardia. A marked increase in the rate of the heart.

Therapeutic. Relating to the science and art of treating people. Therapy may be in the form of medical or surgical treatment, but also involves personal approaches, such as listening, counselling or providing the right environment in which a person feels comfortable and safe.

Thrombosis. The formation of a blood clot (thrombus) on the lining of an artery or vain which may partially or completely block the blood flow through it.

Thrush. An infection due to the yeast-like fungus *candida albicans*. Common sites of infection include the vagina and mouth.

Toxin. Any poisonous compound. Toxins may be released by bacteria multiplying in the body in an infection.

Tranquilliser (see also Medication and Sedation). Medicines that allay anxiety and have a calming effect on the person. They may also prevent them from feeling pain.

Trauma. A wound or injury. Emotional trauma such as bereavement can give rise to mental illness.

Tumour. A lump or swelling in the body. It may be benign or malignant (cancer).

Ulcer. A persistent break in the surface of the skin or the lining of a body cavity (like the stomach).

Ureters. The tubes which drain urine from the kidneys into the bladder.

Urethra. The tube which carries urine from the bladder to the outside.

Urinary tract infection (UTI). An infection that affects the bladder or the urethra.

Varicose veins. A condition, usually of the lower leg, in which the veins are swollen and may be twisted due to structural changes in the walls or valves of the vessels. These veins have difficulty returning blood back to the heart. Knocks to varicose veins commonly cause leg ulcers in older people.

Vascular. Relating to blood vessels, usually arteries or veins.

Venepuncture. The act of puncturing a vein to draw off blood, usually for the purpose of investigation and diagnosis.

Vertigo. A feeling of dizziness accompanied by a feeling that either oneself or one's surroundings are spinning.

Withdrawal (from drugs, alcohol). The physical and mental symptoms experienced by a person when stopping alcohol or drugs that their body has come to depend upon.

Index